Super Easy DASH Diet Cookbook for Beginners

2000+ Days of Flavorful Low-Sodium DASH Diet Recipes, Plus a 30-Day Meal Plan to Promote Wellness, Support Heart Health, and Maintain Healthy Weight

Indulge in Wellness: Where Flavor Meets Healthful Living

Andrew Moore

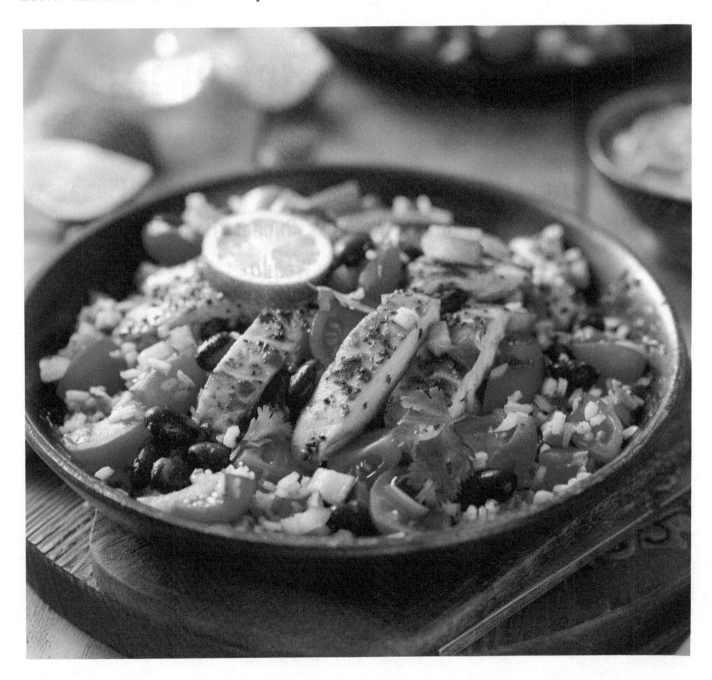

TABLE OF CONTENTS

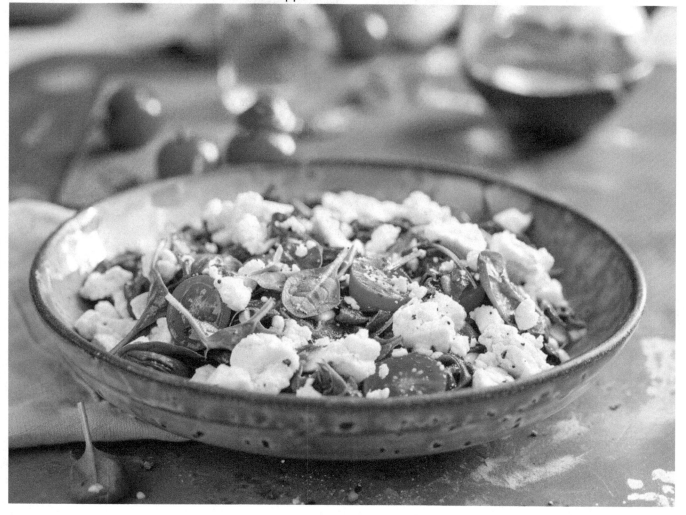

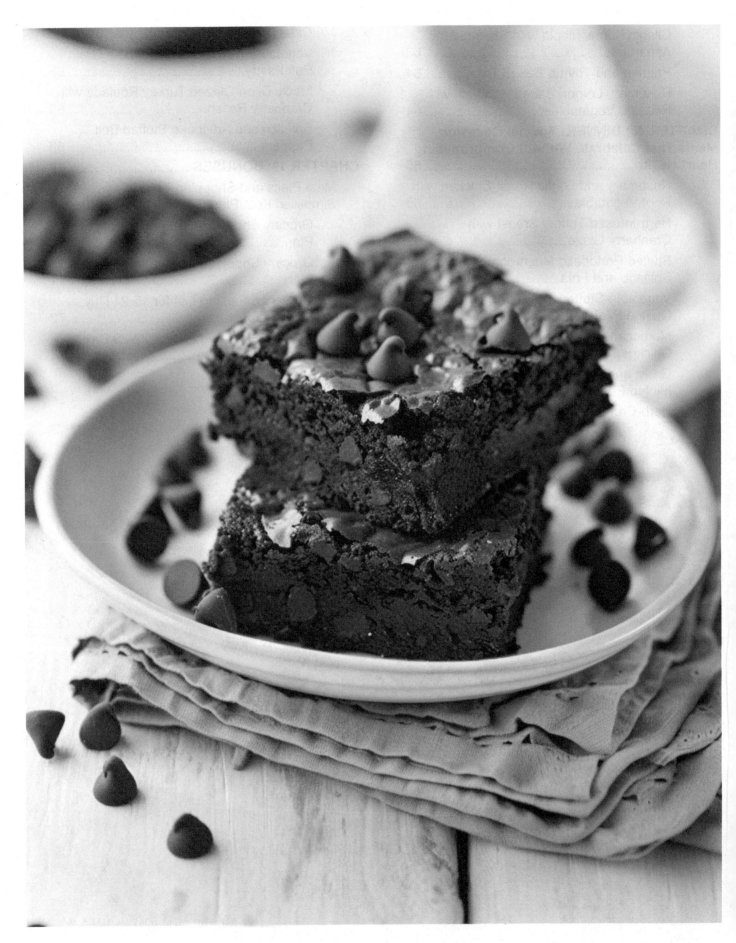

INTRODUCTION

Dear readers,

Andrew Moore, an acclaimed chef and nutrition expert, brings his passion for heart-healthy cooking to life in *Super Easy DASH Diet Cookbook for Beginners.* Known for his innovative approach to creating delicious meals that support wellness, Andrew has crafted a cookbook designed for anyone looking to improve their health through balanced, low-sodium eating.

Andrew doesn't just provide recipes; he empowers you with knowledge and practical tools to succeed. Each recipe is thoughtfully developed to align with the proven principles of the DASH (Dietary Approaches to Stop Hypertension) diet, which is widely recognized for reducing blood pressure, supporting heart health, and preventing chronic disease.

This book is more than a collection of meals—it's your guide to sustainable healthy living. Packed with helpful tips, nutritional insights, and meal-prep strategies, Andrew equips you to make lasting changes in your diet without feeling overwhelmed or deprived.

Discover how the DASH diet can lower blood pressure, improve energy levels, aid in weight management, and promote overall wellness.

With Andrew Moore's expertise, you'll discover that eating well doesn't have to be complicated—it can be easy, enjoyable, and life-changing.

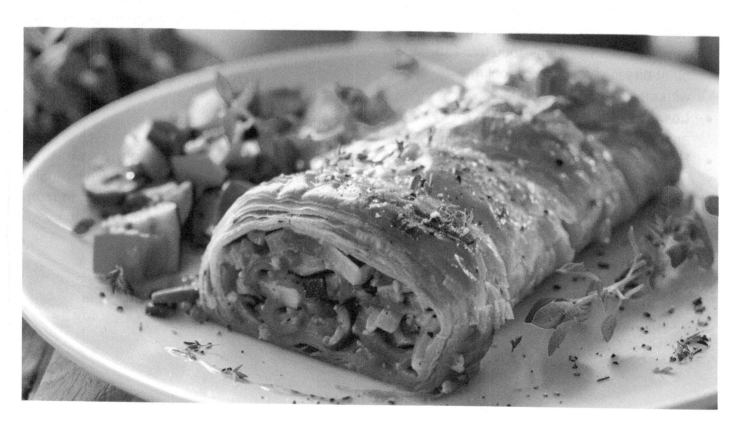

CHAPTER 1: DISCOVERING THE DASH DIET – YOUR PATH TO HEART HEALTH AND VITALITY

Understanding the Science Behind the DASH Diet

The DASH diet was developed by leading researchers to combat hypertension (high blood pressure) and improve overall cardiovascular health. At its core, it emphasizes nutrient-rich foods that are naturally low in sodium and high in essential vitamins, minerals, and fiber.

The primary focus is on:

- **Vegetables and Fruits**: Loaded with antioxidants, vitamins, and potassium, which help balance blood pressure.
- **Whole Grains**: High in fiber, they promote heart health and sustained energy.
- **Lean Proteins**: Think poultry, fish, and plant-based proteins for optimal nutrition without excess saturated fats.
- **Low-Fat Dairy**: A great source of calcium and protein while being heart-friendly.
- **Healthy Fats**: Incorporating nuts, seeds, and oils like olive oil provides essential fatty acids for overall health.

The science is simple: By reducing sodium intake and focusing on nutrient-dense foods, you create a diet that supports heart health and prevents chronic diseases such as hypertension, type 2 diabetes, and obesity.

Understanding Hypertension: The Hidden Dangers, Symptoms, and Causes

Hypertension, commonly known as high blood pressure, is a silent condition that affects millions of people worldwide. It's often called a "silent killer" because it can develop without noticeable symptoms, quietly causing damage to your heart, blood vessels, kidneys, and other vital organs over time.

Blood pressure is the measure of the force your blood exerts on the walls of your arteries. While it's normal for blood pressure to fluctuate throughout the day, consistently high levels can lead to serious health complications, including heart attacks, strokes, and kidney failure.

Symptoms of Hypertension

In many cases, hypertension presents no obvious symptoms, which is why regular check-ups are essential. However, in more severe cases, individuals may experience:

- Headaches
- Shortness of breath
- Nosebleeds
- Dizziness
- Chest pain

These symptoms are not exclusive to hypertension, which makes proper diagnosis critical.

Common Causes of Hypertension

The causes of hypertension can be complex and multifaceted, often influenced by a combination of lifestyle and genetic factors. Common contributors include:

- **High Sodium Intake**: Consuming too much salt can cause your body to retain water, increasing blood pressure.
- **Poor Diet**: Diets high in saturated fats, processed foods, and sugar contribute to weight gain and hypertension.
- **Lack of Physical Activity**: A sedentary lifestyle weakens the heart, making it less efficient in pumping blood.
- **Stress**: Chronic stress can lead to temporary spikes in blood pressure that, over time, become permanent.
- **Family History**: Genetics can play a role, especially if close relatives have had high blood pressure.

The good news? Hypertension is manageable and often preventable with lifestyle changes, and the DASH diet is a proven, science-backed way to lower and control blood pressure naturally.

How the DASH Diet Works: Myths, Facts, and Scientific Evidence

The DASH diet is more than just a meal plan—it's a holistic approach to healthier eating designed to combat hypertension and promote overall well-being. Its success lies in its emphasis on nutrient-dense, unprocessed foods that work together to create a heart-friendly diet.

The Core Principles of the DASH Diet

1. **Focus on Fresh**: The DASH diet prioritizes vegetables, fruits, whole grains, lean proteins, and low-fat dairy. These foods provide essential nutrients like potassium, calcium, and magnesium, which help regulate blood pressure.
2. **Reduce Sodium**: Limiting salt intake is a cornerstone of the DASH diet. Most people consume far more sodium than they need, often from processed foods. The DASH diet encourages natural flavors and low-sodium options.
3. **Balanced Portions**: This diet doesn't eliminate food groups but promotes balanced portions and mindful eating habits.
4. **Healthy Fats**: By replacing saturated and trans fats with heart-healthy fats like those found in nuts, seeds, and olive oil, the DASH diet supports cardiovascular health.

Debunking Common Myths

- **Myth 1: It's Too Restrictive**
  Fact: The DASH diet is incredibly versatile. You'll enjoy a wide variety of delicious foods while making heart-healthy choices.
- **Myth 2: It's Only for People with Hypertension**
  Fact: While designed for managing high blood pressure, the DASH diet benefits anyone seeking a healthier lifestyle.
- **Myth 3: It's Just About Eating Less Salt**
  Fact: While reducing sodium is essential, the DASH diet focuses equally on increasing nutrient-rich foods that support overall health.

The Science Speaks for Itself

The DASH diet isn't just a trend—it's backed by decades of scientific research. Studies consistently show that individuals following the DASH diet experience significant reductions in blood pressure, often comparable to medication. Additional benefits include improved cholesterol levels, better weight management, and a lower risk of chronic diseases such as type 2 diabetes and certain cancers.

Essential Foods for Managing Blood Pressure

The foundation of the DASH diet is built on nutrient-rich foods that work in harmony to lower blood pressure and improve overall health. Incorporating these foods into your daily meals ensures you're not only managing hypertension but also fueling your body with the essential nutrients it needs.

1. Vegetables

Packed with fiber, potassium, and magnesium, vegetables are the cornerstone of the DASH diet. They help regulate blood pressure and support overall heart health. Options like spinach, kale, broccoli, carrots, and bell peppers are excellent choices.

2. Fruits

Fruits provide natural sweetness, antioxidants, and essential vitamins. Bananas, oranges, berries, and melons are rich in potassium, which helps counteract the effects of sodium and supports heart function.

3. Whole Grains

Whole grains such as quinoa, brown rice, oatmeal, and whole wheat bread are high in fiber, which promotes heart health and aids in digestion. These grains also help keep you feeling full and energized throughout the day.

4. Lean Proteins

Poultry, fish, and plant-based proteins like beans, lentils, and tofu are staples of the DASH diet. These options are low in saturated fats and provide high-quality protein to maintain muscle and overall health.

5. Low-Fat Dairy

Dairy products like yogurt, milk, and cheese provide calcium and protein without the excess saturated fat. Opt for low-fat or non-fat versions to maximize heart benefits.

6. Healthy Fats

Fats from sources like olive oil, avocados, nuts, and seeds are essential for heart health. They help reduce bad cholesterol (LDL) while increasing good cholesterol (HDL).

Ingredient Substitution Guide: Healthy Swaps for Your Favorite Dishes

Adopting the DASH diet doesn't mean giving up your favorite dishes. With a few creative substitutions, you can enjoy familiar flavors while sticking to the principles of the DASH diet.

- **Swap Salt with Herbs and Spices**: Use garlic, onion powder, paprika, cumin, basil, oregano, or fresh herbs like cilantro and parsley to enhance flavor naturally.

- **Replace White Rice with Quinoa or Brown Rice**: These options are higher in fiber and provide more nutrients.
- **Use Whole-Grain Pasta Instead of Regular Pasta**: Whole-grain versions are richer in fiber and more filling.
- **Opt for Greek Yogurt Instead of Sour Cream**: Greek yogurt offers creaminess with added protein and less fat.
- **Choose Olive Oil Over Butter**: Olive oil is heart-healthy and versatile in cooking.
- **Replace Processed Snacks with Fresh Alternatives**: Swap chips for homemade popcorn, raw nuts, or sliced vegetables with a low-fat dip.
- **Use Unsweetened Applesauce in Baking**: This can replace sugar or oil for a healthier alternative in cakes and muffins.

These simple swaps allow you to enjoy delicious meals while keeping your heart and health in focus.

Navigating Sodium: Tips for Reducing Salt Without Sacrificing Flavor

One of the key principles of the DASH diet is limiting sodium intake to support healthy blood pressure. However, reducing salt doesn't mean sacrificing taste. Here are practical strategies to keep your meals flavorful and satisfying:

1. Cook from Scratch

Processed and pre-packaged foods are the biggest culprits when it comes to hidden sodium. Preparing meals at home gives you complete control over the ingredients.

2. Explore Natural Flavor Enhancers

Acidic ingredients like lemon juice, lime juice, and vinegar add brightness to dishes, enhancing flavor without the need for salt.

3. Rely on Herbs and Spices

Fresh herbs like parsley, thyme, rosemary, and dill, along with dried spices like paprika, turmeric, and chili powder, can elevate the taste of any dish.

4. Use Low-Sodium Alternatives

Choose low-sodium versions of broths, canned goods, and condiments. These products are widely available and make a noticeable difference in sodium intake.

5. Gradual Reduction

If you're accustomed to salty foods, start reducing salt gradually. Your palate will adapt over time, making lower-sodium dishes just as enjoyable.

6. Get Creative with Textures

Adding contrasting textures, like crunchy nuts or creamy avocado, can make a dish feel more satisfying and flavorful, even with less salt.

7. Read Labels

When shopping, check the sodium content of packaged foods. Aim for products with less than 140 mg of sodium per serving, as these are considered low-sodium.

With planning, mindfulness, and creativity, you can stick to the principles of the DASH diet while savoring every bite. Together, we'll turn these strategies into actionable habits that keep you inspired and motivated on your journey to better health!

CHAPTER 2: 30-DAY MEAL PLAN

Day	Breakfast	Lunch	Snack	Dinner
Day 1	Quinoa Tropical Mango Coconut Porridge - p.15	Tuscan White Bean Minestrone - p.29	Greek Yogurt Parfait with Fresh Fruits - p.43	Herb-Crusted Baked Cod with Lemon Zest - p.62
Day 2	Avocado and Egg Breakfast Bowl - p.20	Lentil and Vegetable Stuffed Eggplant - p.36	Almond & Date Energy Balls - p.44	Spinach and Artichoke Stuffed Bell Peppers - p.69
Day 3	Whole Wheat Blueberry Pancakes - p.21	Grilled Chicken and Quinoa Salad - p.38	Zesty Lemon Herb Tzatziki with Zucchini Chips - p.47	Garlic and Dill Salmon Fillets - p.62
Day 4	Citrus Kale and Orange Smoothie - p.27	Mushroom and Pea Brown Rice Risotto - p.34	Pumpkin Spice Oatmeal Cookies - p.49	Vegetable-Stuffed Acorn Squash with Quinoa Pilaf - p.66
Day 5	Mediterranean Veggie Omelette - p.18	Whole Wheat Veggie Primavera Pasta - p.32	Trail Mix Power Clusters - p.44	Garlic and Herb Roasted Lamb with Minted Pea Puree - p.67
Day 6	Steel-Cut Oat Maple Pecan Pumpkin Porridge - p.15	Moroccan Chickpea and Spinach Soup - p.30	Nutty Quinoa Energy Bars - p.45	Mushroom and Spinach Whole Wheat Lasagna - p.61
Day 7	Southwest Egg Muffins - p.20	Herbed Chicken and Farro Pilaf - p.39	Dark Chocolate Avocado Brownies - p.51	Spiced Shrimp and Vegetable Skewers - p.63
Day 8	Bran and Berry Power Pancakes - p.22	Black Bean and Sweet Potato Buddha Bowl - p.35	Apple Cinnamon Oat Bars - p.45	Maple Dijon Glazed Turkey Roulade with Cranberry Relish - p.69
Day 9	Savory Spinach and Mushroom Oat Porridge - p.17	Barley and Mushroom Soup - p.31	Roasted Red Pepper Hummus with Veggie Sticks - p.46	Herb-Infused Turkey Breast with Cranberry Glaze - p.65
Day 10	Spinach and Feta Egg White Scramble - p.18	Lemon Herb Farro Pasta Salad - p.33	Banana Oatmeal Cookies - p.48	Stuffed Portobello Mushrooms with Spinach and Feta - p.66
Day 11	Almond Flour Lemon Waffles - p.23	Chickpea and Spinach Stuffed Peppers - p.35	Spicy Black Bean Salsa with Whole-Grain Chips - p.47	Cilantro Lime Tilapia with Steamed Asparagus - p.63
Day 12	Tomato Basil Poached Eggs - p.19	Vegetable and Lentil Shepherd's Pie - p.36	Mixed Berry Sorbet - p.55	Cauliflower and Chickpea Tikka Masala - p.61
Day 13	Pumpkin Spice Whole Wheat Muffins - p.23	Grilled Turkey and Avocado Power Bowl - p.38	Raspberry Lemon Tartlets - p.51	Rosemary and Garlic Roast Chicken with Root Vegetables - p.65
Day 14	Mixed Berry and Flaxseed Smoothie - p.28	Creamy Cauliflower and Broccoli Risotto - p.32	Zesty Lemon Herb Tzatziki with Baked Zucchini Chips - p.47	Paprika and Thyme Baked Trout - p.64
Day 15	Savory Spinach and Mushroom Crepes - p.25	Spicy Kidney Bean and Veggie Stir-Fry - p.37	Peach and Almond Crisp - p.50	Herb-Crusted Pork Tenderloin with Apple Cider Reduction - p.68
Day 16	Buckwheat Blueberry Banana Nut Crunch - p.16	Moroccan Chickpea and Spinach Soup - p.30	Cranberry Orange Whole Wheat Muffins - p.53	Spaghetti Squash with Tomato Basil and Spinach - p.60

Day	Breakfast	Lunch	Snack	Dinner
Day 17	Avocado Lime Green Smoothie - p.27	Roasted Vegetable and Barley Pasta - p.34	Lemon Poppy Seed Whole Wheat Scones - p.53	Spinach and Artichoke Stuffed Bell Peppers - p.69
Day 18	Apple Cinnamon Whole Grain Muffins - p.22	Chicken and Black Bean Fiesta Bowl - p.40	Strawberry Basil Gelée - p.55	Balsamic Chicken and Roasted Veggies - p.41
Day 19	Veggie-Packed Breakfast Quinoa Bowl - p.24	Tuscan White Bean Minestrone - p.29	Greek Yogurt Parfait with Fresh Fruits - p.43	Mushroom and Spinach Whole Wheat Lasagna - p.61
Day 20	Cauliflower and Chickpea Herb Bake - p.26	Mushroom and Pea Brown Rice Risotto - p.34	Chia Seed Pudding with Berries - p.48	Garlic and Dill Salmon Fillets - p.62
Day 21	Spinach Apple Ginger Smoothie - p.28	Tuscan White Bean Minestrone - p.29	Banana Walnut Bread - p.54	Lemon Garlic Turkey and Spinach Salad - p.40
Day 22	Hearty Bean and Veggie Breakfast Stew - p.24	Chickpea and Spinach Stuffed Peppers - p.35	Blueberry Almond Muffins - p.50	Vegetable Wellington with Whole Grain Puff Pastry - p.68
Day 23	Berry and Chia Seed Breakfast Tart - p.25	Moroccan Chickpea and Spinach Soup - p.30	Dark Chocolate Avocado Brownies - p.51	Herb-Crusted Pork Tenderloin with Apple Cider Reduction - p.68
Day 24	Lemon Almond Waffles - p.23	Chicken and Vegetable Quinoa - p.42	Zesty Lemon Herb Tzatziki with Baked Zucchini Chips - p.47	Spinach and Artichoke Stuffed Bell Peppers - p.69
Day 25	Mushroom and Herb Frittata - p.19	Barley and Mushroom Soup - p.31	Mixed Berry Sorbet - p.55	Moroccan Vegetable and Chickpea Tart - p.67
Day 26	Whole Wheat Blueberry Pancakes - p.21	Lemon Herb Farro Pasta Salad - p.33	Greek Yogurt Parfait with Fresh Fruits - p.43	Garlic and Dill Salmon Fillets - p.62
Day 27	Steel-Cut Oat Maple Pecan Pumpkin Porridge - p.15	Chickpea and Spinach Stuffed Peppers - p.35	Peach and Almond Crisp - p.50	Herb-Crusted Pork Tenderloin with Apple Cider Reduction - p.68
Day 28	Spinach Apple Ginger Smoothie - p.28	Whole Wheat Veggie Primavera Pasta - p.32	Lemon Poppy Seed Whole Wheat Scones - p.53	Garlic and Herb Roasted Lamb with Minted Pea Puree - p.67
Day 29	Quinoa Tropical Mango Coconut Porridge - p.15	Roasted Vegetable and Barley Pasta - p.34	Cranberry Orange Whole Wheat Muffins - p.53	Vegetable-Stuffed Acorn Squash with Quinoa Pilaf - p.66
Day 30	Almond Flour Lemon Waffles - p.23	Spicy Kidney Bean and Veggie Stir-Fry - p.37	Raspberry Lemon Tartlets - p.51	Rosemary and Garlic Roast Chicken with Root Vegetables - p.65

Note: The 30-day meal plan featured in this book is designed to be a versatile guide and a source of culinary inspiration. The provided caloric and macronutrient values for each recipe are approximate and may vary depending on portion sizes and the specific ingredients you choose. Our meal plan emphasizes a balanced variety of meals, focusing on nutrient-rich proteins and healthy fats while keeping carbohydrates low, aligning with the principles of a ketogenic lifestyle. This approach allows you to maintain a nutritious and enjoyable diet without sacrificing flavor or satisfaction.

If the portion sizes or calorie counts don't align perfectly with your individual dietary requirements, feel free to make adjustments. You can scale the portions up or down to better fit your health objectives and personal preferences. This cookbook is crafted to encourage flexibility and spark creativity in the kitchen, empowering you to create meals that are as unique as your journey to health and wellness!

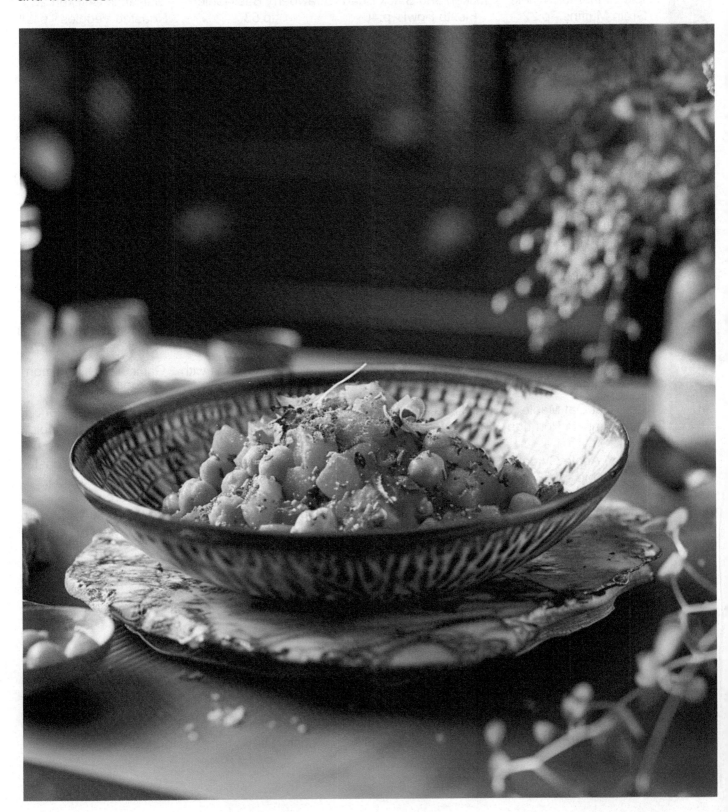

CHAPTER 3: BREAKFASTS: Vibrant Morning Porridges With Fresh Fruits And Vegetables

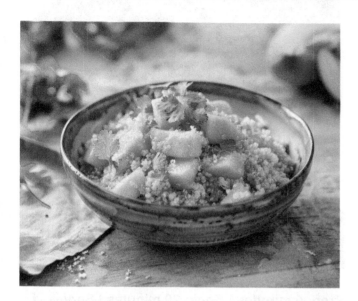

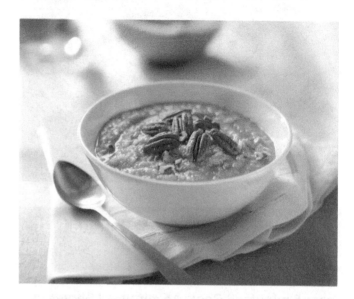

Quinoa Tropical Mango Coconut Porridge

Prep: 5 minutes | Cook: 15 minutes | Serves: 1

Ingredients:

- 1/4 cup quinoa (45g)
- 1/2 cup light coconut milk (120 ml)
- 1/4 cup water (60 ml)
- 1/4 cup diced fresh mango (40g)
- 1 tbsp shredded coconut, unsweetened (7g)
- 1 tsp low carb sweetener, optional (5g)
- 1/4 tsp ground cinnamon (1g)

Instructions:

1. Rinse quinoa under cold water. In a small saucepan, bring quinoa, coconut milk, and water to a boil.
2. Reduce heat, cover, and simmer for 12-15 minutes until quinoa is tender.
3. Stir in diced mango, shredded coconut, and cinnamon. Cook for an additional 2 minutes.
4. Serve warm and garnish with extra mango and coconut if desired.

Nutritional Facts (Per Serving): Calories: 400 | Fat: 11g | Carbs: 30g | Fiber: 8g | Sugars: 11g | Protein: 16g | Sodium: 350 mg

Steel-Cut Oat Maple Pecan Pumpkin Porridge

Prep: 5 minutes | Cook: 20 minutes | Serves: 1

Ingredients:

- 1/4 cup steel-cut oats (45g)
- 1 cup water (240 ml)
- 1/4 cup pumpkin puree (60g)
- 1 tbsp chopped pecans (8g)
- 1 tsp maple syrup (5 ml)
- 1/4 tsp ground cinnamon (1g)
- 1/8 tsp ground nutmeg (0.5g)
- Pinch of salt

Instructions:

1. In a small saucepan, bring water to a boil. Stir in oats, reduce heat, and simmer for 15-20 minutes until tender.
2. Stir in pumpkin puree, maple syrup, cinnamon, nutmeg, and salt. Cook for another 2 minutes until warmed through.
3. Serve topped with chopped pecans.

Nutritional Facts (Per Serving): Calories: 400 | Fat: 13g | Carbs: 28g | Fiber: 7g | Sugars: 11g | Protein: 15g | Sodium: 300 mg

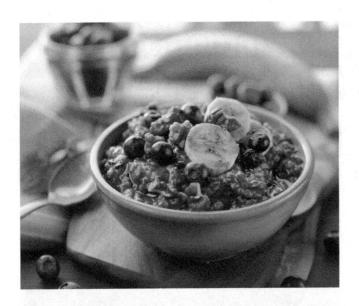

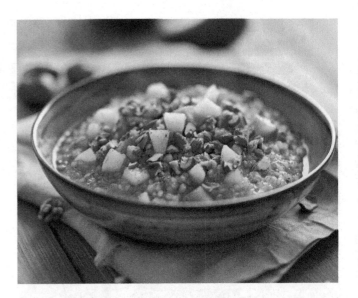

Buckwheat Blueberry Banana Nut Crunch

Prep: 5 minutes | Cook: 15 minutes | Serves: 1

Ingredients:

- 1/4 cup buckwheat groats (45g)
- 1/2 cup water (120 ml)
- 1/4 cup blueberries (35g)
- 1/2 banana, sliced (50g)
- 1 tbsp chopped walnuts (8g)
- 1 tsp low carb sweetener (5g)
- 1/4 tsp ground cinnamon (1g)

Instructions:

1. In a small saucepan, bring water to a boil and add buckwheat. Reduce heat and simmer for 10-12 minutes until tender.
2. Stir in blueberries, banana, sweetener, and cinnamon. Cook for another 2-3 minutes.
3. Top with chopped walnuts and serve warm.

Nutritional Facts (Per Serving): Calories: 400 | Fat: 11g | Carbs: 30g | Fiber: 8g | Sugars: 12g | Protein: 16g | Sodium: 300 mg

Amaranth Spiced Pear and Hazelnut Porridge

Prep: 5 minutes | Cook: 20 minutes | Serves: 1

Ingredients:

- 1/4 cup amaranth (45g)
- 1 cup water (240 ml)
- 1/4 cup diced pear (40g)
- 1 tbsp chopped hazelnuts (8g)
- 1/2 tsp low carb sweetener (2.5g)
- 1/4 tsp ground cardamom (1g)
- Pinch of salt

Instructions:

1. In a small saucepan, bring water to a boil. Add amaranth, reduce heat, and simmer for 15-20 minutes until creamy.
2. Stir in diced pear, sweetener, cardamom, and salt. Cook for another 2 minutes.
3. Top with chopped hazelnuts and serve warm.

Nutritional Facts (Per Serving): Calories: 400 | Fat: 13g | Carbs: 28g | Fiber: 7g | Sugars: 11g | Protein: 15g | Sodium: 300 mg

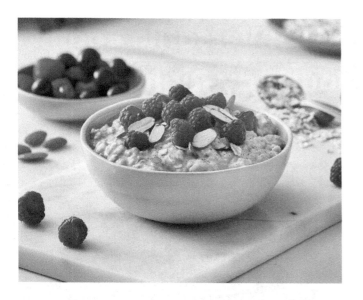

Oatmeal Berry Almond Bliss

Prep: 5 minutes | Cook: 10 minutes | Serves: 1

Ingredients:

- 1/2 cup rolled oats (45g)
- 1 cup water (240 ml)
- 1/4 cup mixed berries (35g)
- 1 tbsp almond butter (16g)
- 1 tsp low carb sweetener (5g)
- 1 tbsp sliced almonds (8g)
- 1/4 tsp ground cinnamon (1g)

Instructions:

1. In a small saucepan, bring water to a boil. Add oats and cook on low heat for 5-7 minutes, stirring occasionally.
2. Stir in almond butter, cinnamon, and sweetener, then cook for another 2-3 minutes until creamy.
3. Top with berries and sliced almonds. Serve warm.

Nutritional Facts (Per Serving): Calories: 400 | Fat: 12g | Carbs: 29g | Fiber: 8g | Sugars: 11g | Protein: 16g | Sodium: 300 mg

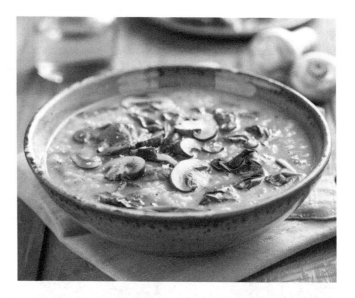

Savory Spinach and Mushroom Oat Porridge

Prep: 5 minutes | Cook: 15 minutes | Serves: 1

Ingredients:

- 1/2 cup rolled oats (45g)
- 1 cup water (240 ml)
- 1/2 cup fresh spinach, chopped (30g)
- 1/4 cup mushrooms, sliced (25g)
- 1 tbsp grated Parmesan cheese (5g)
- 1/2 tsp olive oil (2.5 ml)
- 1/4 tsp garlic powder (1g)
- Pinch of salt and pepper

Instructions:

1. In a small saucepan, heat olive oil and sauté mushrooms until soft, about 3-4 minutes.
2. Add water and oats, then bring to a boil. Reduce heat and simmer for 5-7 minutes until oats are tender.
3. Stir in spinach, Parmesan, garlic powder, salt, and pepper. Cook for another 2-3 minutes until spinach is wilted.
4. Serve warm, garnished with additional Parmesan if desired.

Nutritional Facts (Per Serving): Calories: 400 | Fat: 11g | Carbs: 27g | Fiber: 7g | Sugars: 10g | Protein: 17g | Sodium: 350 mg

CHAPTER 4: BREAKFASTS: Versatile Egg Recipes To Start Your Day Right

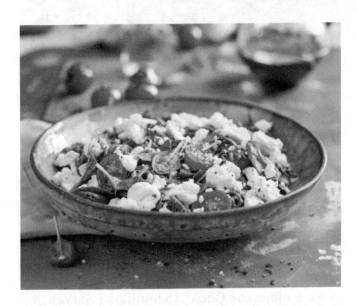

Spinach and Feta Egg White Scramble

Prep: 5 minutes | Cook: 10 minutes | Serves: 1

Ingredients:

- 1 cup egg whites (240 ml)
- 1/2 cup fresh spinach, chopped (30g)
- 1/4 cup crumbled feta cheese (30g)
- 1/4 cup cherry tomatoes, halved (40g)
- 1 tsp olive oil (5 ml)
- Salt and pepper to taste

Instructions:

1. In a skillet, heat olive oil over medium heat. Add spinach and cherry tomatoes, cooking until spinach is wilted, about 2 minutes.
2. Pour in egg whites and cook, stirring frequently, until set.
3. Stir in feta cheese, salt, and pepper, and cook for another minute. Serve warm.

Nutritional Facts (Per Serving): Calories: 400 | Fat: 12g | Carbs: 8g | Fiber: 7g | Sugars: 10g | Protein: 18g | Sodium: 370 mg

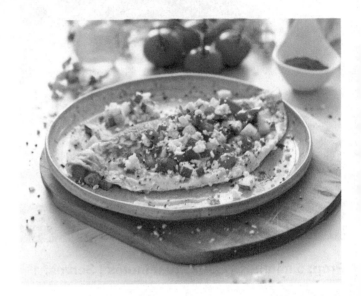

Mediterranean Veggie Omelette

Prep: 5 minutes | Cook: 10 minutes | Serves: 1

Ingredients:

- 2 large eggs (100g)
- 1/4 cup diced bell pepper (30g)
- 1/4 cup diced zucchini (30g)
- 1 tbsp crumbled feta cheese (15g)
- 1 tsp olive oil (5 ml)
- 1/4 tsp dried oregano (1g)
- Salt and pepper to taste

Instructions:

1. In a skillet, heat olive oil over medium heat. Add bell pepper and zucchini, cooking until softened, about 3 minutes.
2. In a bowl, whisk eggs with oregano, salt, and pepper.
3. Pour eggs into the skillet and cook until edges begin to set, then sprinkle feta on top. Fold and cook until eggs are fully set. Serve warm.

Nutritional Facts (Per Serving): Calories: 400 | Fat: 13g | Carbs: 9g | Fiber: 7g | Sugars: 10g | Protein: 17g | Sodium: 350 mg

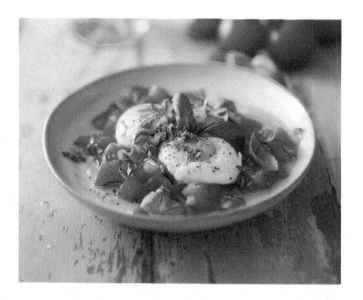

Tomato Basil Poached Eggs

Prep: 5 minutes | Cook: 10 minutes | Serves: 1

Ingredients:

- 2 large eggs (100g)
- 1/2 cup diced tomatoes (90g)
- 1/4 cup fresh basil, chopped (10g)
- 1/4 cup water (60 ml)
- 1 tsp olive oil (5 ml)
- Salt and pepper to taste

Instructions:

1. In a skillet, heat olive oil over medium heat. Add diced tomatoes and cook for 2-3 minutes until softened.
2. Add water and bring to a simmer. Carefully crack eggs into the skillet, season with salt and pepper, and poach until whites are set, about 4-5 minutes.
3. Sprinkle with fresh basil and serve warm.

Nutritional Facts (Per Serving): Calories: 400 | Fat: 12g | Carbs: 8g | Fiber: 7g | Sugars: 10g | Protein: 17g | Sodium: 360 mg

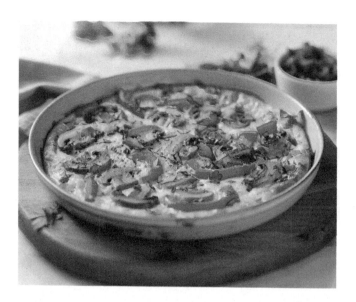

Mushroom and Herb Frittata

Prep: 5 minutes | Cook: 15 minutes | Serves: 1

Ingredients:

- 2 large eggs (100g)
- 1/2 cup mushrooms, sliced (50g)
- 1/4 cup diced bell pepper (30g)
- 1 tbsp fresh parsley, chopped (5g)
- 1 tbsp grated Parmesan cheese (5g)
- 1 tsp olive oil (5 ml)
- Salt and pepper to taste

Instructions:

1. Preheat oven to 375°F (190°C).
2. In an oven-safe skillet, heat olive oil over medium heat. Sauté mushrooms and bell pepper until softened, about 3-4 minutes.
3. In a bowl, whisk eggs, parsley, Parmesan, salt, and pepper. Pour over vegetables in the skillet.
4. Transfer skillet to the oven and bake for 8-10 minutes until eggs are set. Serve warm.

Nutritional Facts (Per Serving): Calories: 400 | Fat: 13g | Carbs: 9g | Fiber: 7g | Sugars: 10g | Protein: 16g | Sodium: 350 mg

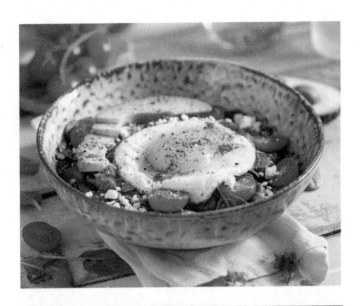

Avocado and Egg Breakfast Bowl

Prep: 5 minutes | Cook: 10 minutes | Serves: 1

Ingredients:

- 1 large egg (50g)
- 1/2 avocado, sliced (70g)
- 1/2 cup cherry tomatoes, halved (75g)
- 1/4 cup baby spinach (15g)
- 1 tbsp feta cheese, crumbled (15g)
- 1 tsp olive oil (5 ml)
- Salt and pepper to taste

Instructions:

1. In a small skillet, heat olive oil over medium heat. Crack the egg into the skillet and cook until the whites are set.
2. In a bowl, arrange avocado, tomatoes, and spinach. Top with the cooked egg and sprinkle with feta, salt, and pepper. Serve warm.

Nutritional Facts (Per Serving): Calories: 400 | Fat: 13g | Carbs: 15g | Fiber: 8g | Sugars: 10g | Protein: 17g | Sodium: 350 mg

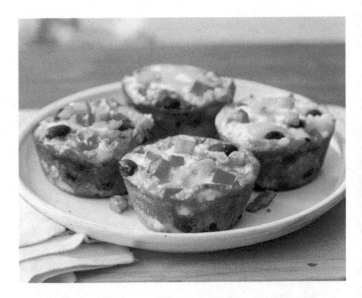

Southwest Egg Muffins

Prep: 10 minutes | Cook: 20 minutes | Serves: 1

Ingredients:

- 2 large eggs (100g)
- 1/4 cup black beans, drained and rinsed (40g)
- 1/4 cup diced bell pepper (30g)
- 1 tbsp shredded cheddar cheese (10g)
- 1 tsp low carb sweetener (5g), optional
- 1/4 tsp chili powder (1g)
- Salt and pepper to taste

Instructions:

1. Preheat the oven to 350°F (175°C) and grease a muffin tin.
2. In a bowl, whisk together eggs, black beans, bell pepper, cheese, chili powder, salt, and pepper.
3. Pour the mixture into the prepared muffin tin and bake for 18-20 minutes until eggs are set. Serve warm.

Nutritional Facts (Per Serving): Calories: 400 | Fat: 12g | Carbs: 14g | Fiber: 7g | Sugars: 10g | Protein: 18g | Sodium: 340 mg

CHAPTER 5: BREAKFASTS: Hearty Whole Grain Options: Pancakes, Waffles, And Muffins

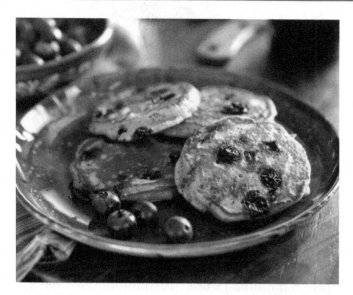

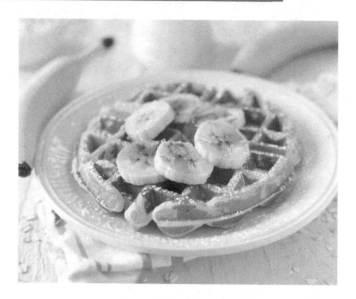

Whole Wheat Blueberry Pancakes

Prep: 5 minutes | Cook: 10 minutes | Serves: 1

Ingredients:

- 1/4 cup whole wheat flour (30g)
- 1/4 cup blueberries (35g)
- 1/4 cup unsweetened almond milk (60 ml)
- 1 large egg (50g)
- 1/2 tsp low carb sweetener (2.5g)
- 1/4 tsp baking powder (1g)
- 1/4 tsp vanilla extract (1 ml)
- 1/4 tsp cinnamon (1g)

Instructions:

1. In a bowl, whisk together flour, baking powder, and cinnamon. Add egg, almond milk, vanilla, and sweetener, stirring until smooth.
2. Gently fold in blueberries.
3. Heat a non-stick skillet over medium heat. Pour batter onto the skillet, forming small pancakes, and cook for 2-3 minutes per side until golden. Serve warm.

Nutritional Facts (Per Serving): Calories: 400 | Fat: 12g | Carbs: 28g | Fiber: 8g | Sugars: 11g | Protein: 16g | Sodium: 350 mg

Banana Oatmeal Protein Waffles

Prep: 5 minutes | Cook: 10 minutes | Serves: 1

Ingredients:

- 1/4 cup rolled oats (25g)
- 1/2 banana, mashed (50g)
- 1 large egg (50g)
- 1/4 cup low-fat Greek yogurt (60g)
- 1 tbsp protein powder (10g)
- 1/4 tsp baking powder (1g)
- 1/4 tsp cinnamon (1g)
- 1/4 tsp vanilla extract (1 ml)

Instructions:

1. In a blender, combine oats, banana, egg, Greek yogurt, protein powder, baking powder, cinnamon, and vanilla. Blend until smooth.
2. Preheat a waffle iron and lightly grease if needed. Pour the batter into the waffle iron and cook according to the manufacturer's instructions until golden.
3. Serve warm, topped with extra banana slices if desired.

Nutritional Facts (Per Serving): Calories: 400 | Fat: 11g | Carbs: 30g | Fiber: 7g | Sugars: 10g | Protein: 18g | Sodium: 330 mg

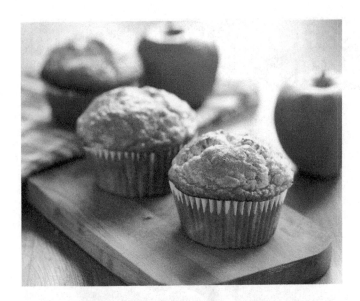

Apple Cinnamon Whole Grain Muffins

Prep: 10 minutes | Cook: 20 minutes | Serves: 1

Ingredients:

- 1/4 cup whole wheat flour (30g)
- 1/4 cup grated apple (30g)
- 1 tbsp rolled oats (8g)
- 1 large egg (50g)
- 1 tbsp low-fat Greek yogurt (15g)
- 1/2 tsp low carb sweetener (2.5g)
- 1/4 tsp baking powder (1g)
- 1/4 tsp cinnamon (1g)
- 1/4 tsp vanilla extract (1 ml)

Instructions:

1. Preheat oven to 350°F (175°C) and line a muffin tin with a paper liner.
2. In a bowl, combine flour, oats, baking powder, and cinnamon.
3. In another bowl, whisk egg, yogurt, sweetener, and vanilla, then fold in grated apple.
4. Combine wet and dry ingredients, then pour into muffin tin.
5. Bake for 20 minutes or until a toothpick comes out clean. Serve warm.

Nutritional Facts (Per Serving): Calories: 400 | Fat: 12g | Carbs: 28g | Fiber: 8g | Sugars: 11g | Protein: 16g | Sodium: 350 mg

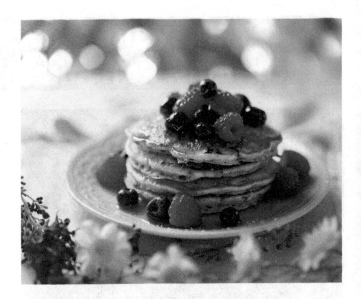

Bran and Berry Power Pancakes

Prep: 5 minutes | Cook: 10 minutes | Serves: 1

Ingredients:

- 1/4 cup bran flakes (25g)
- 1/4 cup mixed berries (35g)
- 1/4 cup almond milk (60 ml)
- 1 large egg (50g)
- 1 tbsp whole wheat flour (8g)
- 1/2 tsp low carb sweetener (2.5g)
- 1/4 tsp baking powder (1g)
- 1/4 tsp vanilla extract (1 ml)

Instructions:

1. In a bowl, combine bran flakes, flour, baking powder, and sweetener.
2. Add egg, almond milk, and vanilla, mixing until smooth, then fold in berries.
3. Heat a non-stick skillet over medium heat. Pour batter onto the skillet, forming pancakes, and cook for 2-3 minutes per side.
4. Serve warm, topped with extra berries if desired.

Nutritional Facts (Per Serving): Calories: 400 | Fat: 11g | Carbs: 29g | Fiber: 8g | Sugars: 10g | Protein: 17g | Sodium: 320 mg

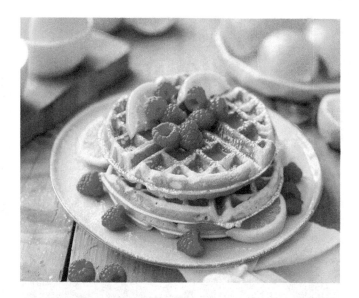

Almond Flour Lemon Waffles

Prep: 5 minutes | Cook: 10 minutes | Serves: 1

Ingredients:

- 1/4 cup almond flour (25g)
- 1 large egg (50g)
- 1 tbsp unsweetened almond milk (15 ml)
- 1 tsp lemon zest (2g)
- 1 tsp low carb sweetener (5g)
- 1/4 tsp baking powder (1g)
- 1/4 tsp vanilla extract (1 ml)

Instructions:

1. In a bowl, whisk together almond flour, baking powder, lemon zest, and sweetener.
2. Add egg, almond milk, and vanilla, stirring until smooth.
3. Preheat a waffle iron and lightly grease if necessary. Pour the batter into the waffle iron and cook until golden.
4. Serve warm with a sprinkle of extra lemon zest if desired.

Nutritional Facts (Per Serving): Calories: 400 | Fat: 12g | Carbs: 14g | Fiber: 8g | Sugars: 10g | Protein: 16g | Sodium: 340 mg

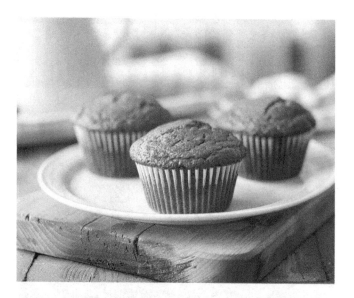

Pumpkin Spice Whole Wheat Muffins

Prep: 10 minutes | Cook: 20 minutes | Serves: 1

Ingredients:

- 1/4 cup whole wheat flour (30g)
- 2 tbsp pumpkin puree (30g)
- 1 large egg (50g)
- 1 tbsp low-fat Greek yogurt (15g)
- 1 tsp low carb sweetener (5g)
- 1/4 tsp baking powder (1g)
- 1/4 tsp pumpkin spice (1g)
- 1/4 tsp vanilla extract (1 ml)

Instructions:

1. Preheat the oven to 350°F (175°C) and line a muffin tin with a paper liner.
2. In a bowl, combine flour, baking powder, and pumpkin spice.
3. In another bowl, whisk egg, pumpkin puree, Greek yogurt, sweetener, and vanilla.
4. Combine wet and dry ingredients, mixing until smooth, then pour into the muffin tin.
5. Bake for 20 minutes or until a toothpick comes out clean. Serve warm.

Nutritional Facts (Per Serving): Calories: 400 | Fat: 11g | Carbs: 28g | Fiber: 8g | Sugars: 11g | Protein: 17g | Sodium: 360 mg

CHAPTER 6: BREAKFASTS: Delightful Weekend Breakfast Ideas That Adhere To The Dash Diet

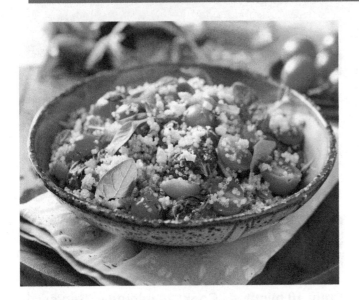

Veggie-Packed Breakfast Quinoa Bowl

Prep: 5 minutes | Cook: 15 minutes | Serves: 1

Ingredients:

- 1/4 cup quinoa (45g)
- 1/2 cup water (120 ml)
- 1/4 cup cherry tomatoes, halved (40g)
- 1/4 cup baby spinach, chopped (15g)
- 1 tbsp feta cheese, crumbled (15g)
- 1 tsp olive oil (5 ml)
- Salt and pepper to taste

Instructions:

1. Rinse quinoa under cold water. In a small saucepan, bring quinoa and water to a boil. Reduce heat, cover, and simmer for 12-15 minutes until quinoa is tender.
2. In a bowl, combine cooked quinoa, cherry tomatoes, spinach, and feta. Drizzle with olive oil, season with salt and pepper, and serve warm.

Nutritional Facts (Per Serving): Calories: 400 | Fat: 12g | Carbs: 28g | Fiber: 8g | Sugars: 10g | Protein: 17g | Sodium: 360 mg

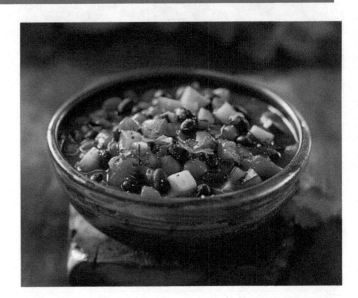

Hearty Bean and Veggie Breakfast Stew

Prep: 5 minutes | Cook: 15 minutes | Serves: 1

Ingredients:

- 1/4 cup canned black beans, rinsed and drained (40g)
- 1/4 cup diced bell pepper (30g)
- 1/4 cup zucchini, diced (30g)
- 1/2 cup low-sodium vegetable broth (120 ml)
- 1 tbsp diced onion (10g)
- 1 tsp olive oil (5 ml)
- 1/4 tsp ground cumin (1g)
- Salt and pepper to taste

Instructions:

1. In a small pot, heat olive oil over medium heat. Sauté onion, bell pepper, and zucchini until softened, about 3-4 minutes.
2. Add black beans, vegetable broth, and cumin. Bring to a simmer and cook for 10 minutes until flavors meld.
3. Season with salt and pepper. Serve warm.

Nutritional Facts (Per Serving): Calories: 400 | Fat: 11g | Carbs: 30g | Fiber: 8g | Sugars: 11g | Protein: 16g | Sodium: 370 mg

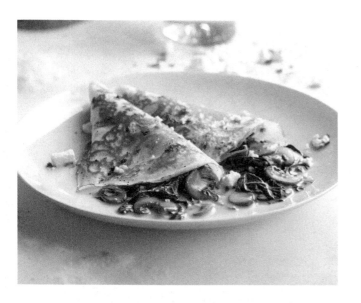

Savory Spinach and Mushroom Crepes

Prep: 10 minutes | Cook: 15 minutes | Serves: 1

Ingredients:

- 1/4 cup whole wheat flour (30g)
- 1 large egg (50g)
- 1/4 cup unsweetened almond milk (60 ml)
- 1/4 cup mushrooms, sliced (30g)
- 1/4 cup fresh spinach, chopped (15g)
- 1 tbsp feta cheese, crumbled (15g)
- 1 tsp olive oil (5 ml)
- Salt and pepper to taste

Instructions:

1. In a bowl, whisk together flour, egg, and almond milk until smooth. Set aside.
2. In a skillet, heat olive oil over medium heat. Sauté mushrooms and spinach until softened, about 3 minutes.
3. Pour a thin layer of batter into a non-stick pan, cook until set, then flip. Fill with spinach, mushrooms, and feta. Fold and serve warm.

Nutritional Facts (Per Serving): Calories: 400 | Fat: 12g | Carbs: 28g | Fiber: 8g | Sugars: 10g | Protein: 17g | Sodium: 360 mg

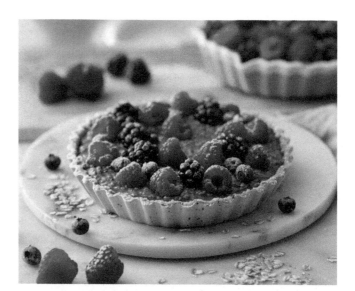

Berry and Chia Seed Breakfast Tart

Prep: 5 minutes | Cook: 10 minutes | Serves: 1

Ingredients:

- 1/4 cup rolled oats (25g)
- 1/4 cup almond milk (60 ml)
- 1/4 cup mixed berries (35g)
- 1 tbsp chia seeds (10g)
- 1 tsp low carb sweetener (5g)
- 1/2 tsp vanilla extract (2 ml)

Instructions:

1. In a small saucepan, combine oats, almond milk, and chia seeds. Cook over medium heat for 5-7 minutes until thickened.
2. Stir in vanilla and sweetener, then pour into a small bowl or tart mold.
3. Top with mixed berries and serve chilled or warm.

Nutritional Facts (Per Serving): Calories: 400 | Fat: 11g | Carbs: 27g | Fiber: 8g | Sugars: 11g | Protein: 15g | Sodium: 300 mg

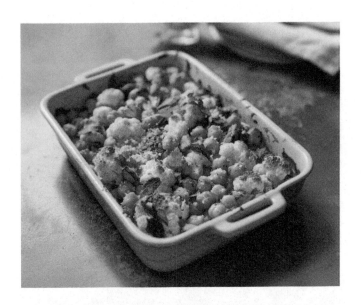

Cauliflower and Chickpea Herb Bake

Prep: 10 minutes | Cook: 30 minutes | Serves: 1

Ingredients:

- 1/2 cup cauliflower florets, chopped (75g)
- 1/4 cup canned chickpeas, rinsed and drained (40g)
- 1 large egg (50g)
- 1 tbsp fresh parsley, chopped (5g)
- 1 tbsp grated Parmesan cheese (5g)
- 1/2 tsp olive oil (2.5 ml)
- 1/4 tsp garlic powder (1g)
- Salt and pepper to taste

Instructions:

1. Preheat the oven to 375°F (190°C) and lightly grease a small baking dish with olive oil.
2. In a bowl, mix cauliflower, chickpeas, parsley, Parmesan, garlic powder, salt, and pepper.
3. Add the egg and mix until well combined. Pour the mixture into the baking dish.
4. Bake for 25-30 minutes, until golden and set. Serve warm.

Nutritional Facts (Per Serving): Calories: 400 | Fat: 12g | Carbs: 26g | Fiber: 8g | Sugars: 10g | Protein: 16g | Sodium: 350 mg

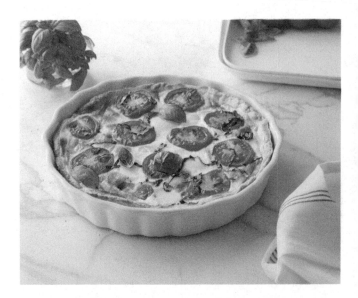

Tomato, Basil, and Mozzarella Quiche

Prep: 10 minutes | Cook: 35 minutes | Serves: 1

Ingredients:

- 1/4 cup cherry tomatoes, halved (40g)
- 1/4 cup fresh basil, chopped (10g)
- 1/4 cup shredded mozzarella cheese (30g)
- 1/4 cup unsweetened almond milk (60 ml)
- 2 large eggs (100g)
- 1/2 tsp olive oil (2.5 ml)
- Salt and pepper to taste

Instructions:

1. Preheat the oven to 375°F (190°C) and grease a small pie dish with olive oil.
2. In a bowl, whisk together eggs, almond milk, salt, and pepper.
3. Add tomatoes, basil, and mozzarella. Pour the mixture into the pie dish.
4. Bake for 30-35 minutes, until set and lightly golden. Serve warm.

Nutritional Facts (Per Serving): Calories: 400 | Fat: 13g | Carbs: 12g | Fiber: 7g | Sugars: 11g | Protein: 18g | Sodium: 370 mg

CHAPTER 7: BREAKFASTS: Refreshing Low-Sugar Smoothies

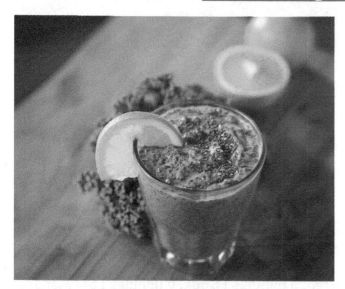

Citrus Kale and Orange Smoothie

Prep: 5 minutes | Cook: 0 minutes | Serves: 1

Ingredients:

- 1 cup kale leaves, chopped (30g)
- 1/2 cup unsweetened almond milk (120 ml)
- 1/2 orange, peeled (75g)
- 1/4 cup Greek yogurt (60g)
- 1 tbsp chia seeds (10g)
- 1 tsp low carb sweetener (5g)
- 1/2 tsp orange zest (1g)

Instructions:

1. In a blender, combine kale, almond milk, orange, Greek yogurt, chia seeds, sweetener, and orange zest.
2. Blend until smooth.
3. Serve immediately.

Nutritional Facts (Per Serving): Calories: 400 | Fat: 12g | Carbs: 27g | Fiber: 8g | Sugars: 11g | Protein: 16g | Sodium: 350 mg

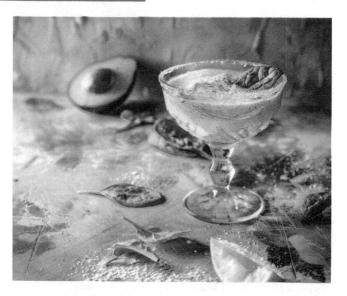

Avocado Lime Green Smoothie

Prep: 5 minutes | Cook: 0 minutes | Serves: 1

Ingredients:

- 1/2 avocado (70g)
- 1 cup spinach leaves (30g)
- 1/2 cup unsweetened coconut water (120 ml)
- 1/4 cup Greek yogurt (60g)
- 1 tbsp lime juice (15 ml)
- 1 tsp low carb sweetener (5g)
- 1/4 tsp lime zest (1g)

Instructions:

1. In a blender, combine avocado, spinach, coconut water, Greek yogurt, lime juice, sweetener, and lime zest.
2. Blend until creamy.
3. Serve immediately.

Nutritional Facts (Per Serving): Calories: 400 | Fat: 13g | Carbs: 25g | Fiber: 8g | Sugars: 10g | Protein: 17g | Sodium: 330 mg

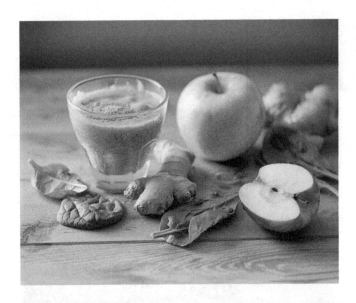

Spinach Apple Ginger Smoothie

Prep: 5 minutes | Cook: 0 minutes | Serves: 1

Ingredients:

- 1 cup fresh spinach (30g)
- 1/2 apple, chopped (75g)
- 1/2 cup unsweetened almond milk (120 ml)
- 1/4 cup Greek yogurt (60g)
- 1 tsp fresh ginger, grated (5g)
- 1 tsp low carb sweetener (5g)
- 1/2 tsp cinnamon (1g)

Instructions:

1. In a blender, combine spinach, apple, almond milk, Greek yogurt, ginger, sweetener, and cinnamon.
2. Blend until smooth.
3. Serve immediately.

Nutritional Facts (Per Serving): Calories: 400 | Fat: 12g | Carbs: 26g | Fiber: 8g | Sugars: 11g | Protein: 16g | Sodium: 330 mg

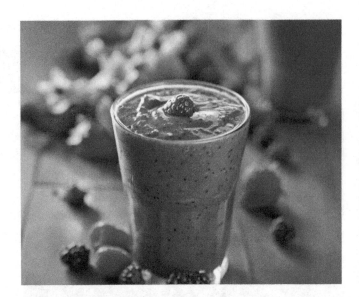

Mixed Berry and Flaxseed Smoothie

Prep: 5 minutes | Cook: 0 minutes | Serves: 1

Ingredients:

- 1/2 cup mixed berries (70g)
- 1/2 cup unsweetened almond milk (120 ml)
- 1/4 cup Greek yogurt (60g)
- 1 tbsp ground flaxseed (7g)
- 1 tsp low carb sweetener (5g)
- 1/4 tsp vanilla extract (1 ml)

Instructions:

1. In a blender, combine mixed berries, almond milk, Greek yogurt, flaxseed, sweetener, and vanilla.
2. Blend until smooth.
3. Serve immediately.

Nutritional Facts (Per Serving): Calories: 400 | Fat: 11g | Carbs: 28g | Fiber: 8g | Sugars: 12g | Protein: 17g | Sodium: 350 mg

CHAPTER 8: LUNCHES: Comforting Soups And Nutrient-Dense Stews

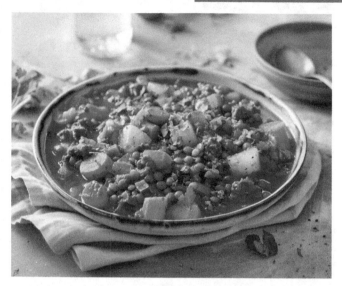

Hearty Lentil and Vegetable Stew

Prep: 15 minutes | Cook: 40 minutes | Serves: 1

Ingredients:

- 1/4 cup dry green lentils (50g)
- 1/2 tbsp olive oil (7g)
- 1/2 cup diced carrots (75g)
- 1/2 cup diced celery (75g)
- 1/2 cup diced onion (75g)
- 1 garlic clove, minced (3g)
- 1/4 cup diced tomatoes (60g)
- 1/2 cup low-sodium vegetable broth (120ml)
- 1/2 tsp dried thyme (0.5g)
- 1/4 tsp dried rosemary (0.3g)
- 1 bay leaf
- Salt and pepper to taste

Instructions:

1. Heat olive oil in a pot over medium heat. Sauté carrots, celery, onion, and garlic until softened, about 5 minutes.
2. Add lentils, diced tomatoes, vegetable broth, thyme, rosemary, bay leaf, salt, and pepper. Bring to a boil, then reduce to simmer.
3. Cook until lentils are tender, about 30 minutes. Remove bay leaf and adjust seasoning.
4. Serve warm.

Nutritional Facts (Per Serving): Calories: 500 | Fat: 5g | Carbs: 30g | Fiber: 8g | Sugars: 12g | Protein: 20g | Sodium: 350mg

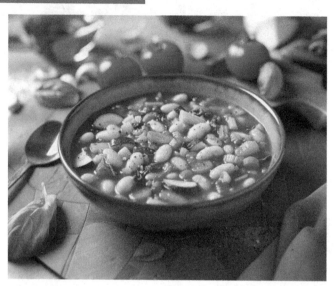

Tuscan White Bean Minestrone

Prep: 15 minutes | Cook: 30 minutes | Serves: 1

Ingredients:

- 1/2 tbsp olive oil (7g)
- 1/4 cup diced carrots (40g)
- 1/4 cup diced celery (40g)
- 1/4 cup diced onion (40g)
- 1 garlic clove, minced (3g)
- 1/2 cup canned white beans, rinsed (75g)
- 1/2 cup chopped zucchini (75g)
- 1/2 cup chopped tomatoes (75g)
- 1/2 cup low-sodium vegetable broth (120ml)
- 1/4 tsp dried basil (0.3g)
- 1/4 tsp dried oregano (0.3g)
- Salt and pepper to taste

Instructions:

1. In a pot, heat olive oil over medium heat. Sauté carrots, celery, onion, and garlic until softened, about 5 minutes.
2. Add white beans, zucchini, tomatoes, vegetable broth, basil, oregano, salt, and pepper. Bring to a boil, then reduce to a simmer.
3. Simmer for about 20 minutes until all vegetables are tender. Serve hot.

Nutritional Facts (Per Serving): Calories: 500 | Fat: 5g | Carbs: 30g | Fiber: 10g | Sugars: 12g | Protein: 20g | Sodium: 300mg

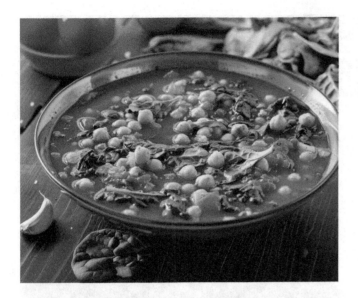

Moroccan Chickpea and Spinach Soup

Prep: 15 minutes | Cook: 30 minutes | Serves: 1

Ingredients:

- 1/2 tbsp olive oil (7g)
- 1/4 cup diced onion (40g)
- 1 garlic clove, minced (3g)
- 1/4 tsp ground cumin (0.5g)
- 1/4 tsp ground coriander (0.5g)
- 1/8 tsp ground cinnamon (0.3g)
- 1/4 cup diced tomatoes (60g)
- 1/2 cup low-sodium vegetable broth (120ml)
- 1/4 cup canned chickpeas, rinsed (40g)
- 1 cup fresh spinach leaves (30g)
- Salt and pepper to taste

Instructions:

1. Heat olive oil in a pot over medium heat. Sauté onion and garlic until soft, about 5 minutes.
2. Add cumin, coriander, and cinnamon; cook for 1 minute.
3. Add tomatoes, broth, and chickpeas. Bring to a boil, then reduce to a simmer.
4. Simmer for 20 minutes. Stir in spinach and cook until wilted, about 2 minutes. Season to taste with salt and pepper.
5. Serve warm.

Nutritional Facts (Per Serving): Calories: 500 | Fat: 5g | Carbs: 30g | Fiber: 9g | Sugars: 12g | Protein: 20g | Sodium: 350mg

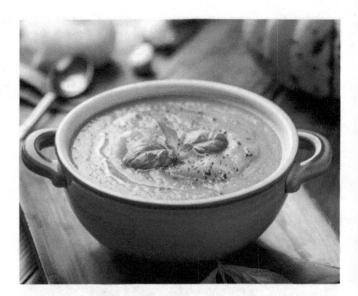

Creamy Butternut Squash and Quinoa Soup

Prep: 15 minutes | Cook: 25 minutes | Serves: 1

Ingredients:

- 1/2 tbsp olive oil (7g)
- 1/2 cup diced butternut squash (75g)
- 1/4 cup diced onion (40g)
- 1 garlic clove, minced (3g)
- 1/4 cup quinoa, rinsed (50g)
- 1/2 cup low-sodium vegetable broth (120ml)
- 1/2 cup unsweetened almond milk (120ml)
- 1/8 tsp ground nutmeg (0.2g)
- Salt and pepper to taste

Instructions:

1. In a pot, heat olive oil over medium heat. Sauté butternut squash, onion, and garlic until softened, about 5 minutes.
2. Add quinoa, vegetable broth, almond milk, and nutmeg. Bring to a boil, then reduce heat to simmer.
3. Simmer until squash is tender and quinoa is cooked, about 20 minutes. Season with salt and pepper to taste.
4. Puree with an immersion blender for a creamy consistency, if desired. Serve warm.

Nutritional Facts (Per Serving): Calories: 500 | Fat: 5g | Carbs: 30g | Fiber: 9g | Sugars: 13g | Protein: 20g | Sodium: 300mg

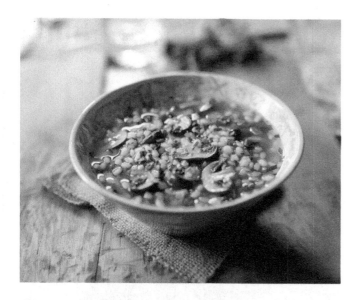

Barley and Mushroom Soup

Prep: 15 minutes | Cook: 40 minutes | Serves: 1

Ingredients:

- 1/2 tbsp olive oil (7g)
- 1/4 cup pearl barley (50g)
- 1/2 cup sliced mushrooms (75g)
- 1/4 cup diced onion (40g)
- 1 garlic clove, minced (3g)
- 1/2 cup low-sodium vegetable broth (120ml)
- 1/2 cup water (120ml)
- 1/4 tsp dried thyme (0.5g)
- Salt and pepper to taste

Instructions:

1. Heat olive oil in a pot over medium heat. Add the mushrooms, onion, and garlic; sauté until soft and fragrant, about 5 minutes, stirring occasionally.
2. Add the barley, stirring to coat it with the oil. Let it cook for 1-2 minutes to enhance its flavor.
3. Pour in the vegetable broth, water, thyme, salt, and pepper. Stir and bring to a boil.
4. Reduce the heat to a simmer. Partially cover the pot and cook, stirring occasionally, until the barley is tender, about 30 minutes.
5. Adjust seasoning if needed.
6. Serve warm.

Nutritional Facts (Per Serving): Calories: 500 | Fat: 5g | Carbs: 30g | Fiber: 9g | Sugars: 12g | Protein: 20g | Sodium: 350mg

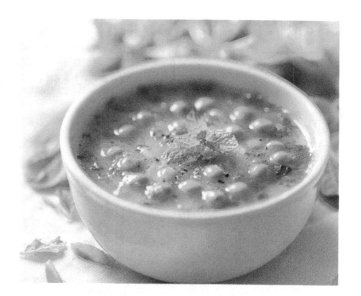

Green Pea and Mint Vegetable Soup

Prep: 10 minutes | Cook: 20 minutes | Serves: 1

Ingredients:

- 1/2 tbsp olive oil (7g)
- 1/2 cup green peas (75g)
- 1/4 cup diced onion (40g)
- 1 garlic clove, minced (3g)
- 1/2 cup low-sodium vegetable broth (120ml)
- 1/2 cup water (120ml)
- 1/4 tsp dried mint (0.5g)
- 1/4 cup fresh spinach (10g)
- Salt and pepper to taste

Instructions:

1. In a pot, heat the olive oil over medium heat. Add the diced onion and minced garlic, and sauté until softened and fragrant, stirring occasionally, about 5 minutes.
2. Add the peas and stir to coat them in the oil.
3. Pour in the broth, water, mint, and spinach. Season with salt and pepper, then bring to a boil.
4. Reduce to a simmer, cover partially, and cook for 10-15 minutes, until peas are tender.
5. Puree with an immersion blender to desired consistency, adjust seasoning if needed, and serve warm.

Nutritional Facts (Per Serving): Calories: 500 | Fat: 5g | Carbs: 30g | Fiber: 10g | Sugars: 12g | Protein: 20g | Sodium: 300mg

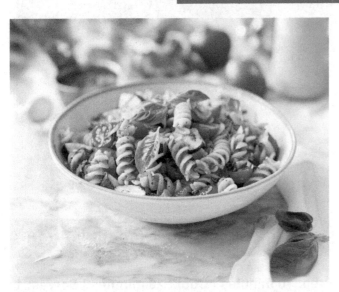

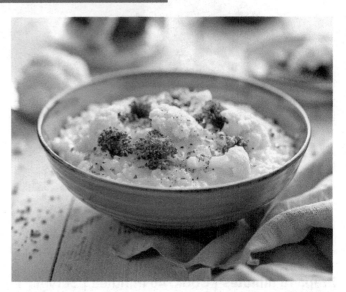

Whole Wheat Veggie Primavera Pasta

Prep: 15 minutes | Cook: 20 minutes | Serves: 1

Ingredients:

- 1/2 cup whole wheat pasta (75g)
- 1/2 tbsp olive oil (7g)
- 1/4 cup diced zucchini (40g)
- 1/4 cup cherry tomatoes, halved (40g)
- 1/4 cup sliced bell pepper (40g)
- 1 garlic clove, minced (3g)
- 1/2 cup fresh spinach (15g)
- 1/4 tsp dried basil (0.5g)
- 1/4 tsp dried oregano (0.5g)
- Salt and pepper to taste

Instructions:

1. Cook pasta according to package instructions. Drain and set aside.

2. Heat olive oil in a pan over medium heat. Sauté zucchini, bell pepper, and garlic until tender, about 5 minutes.

3. Add cherry tomatoes, spinach, basil, and oregano. Cook until spinach is wilted.

4. Toss cooked pasta with vegetable mixture, season with salt and pepper, and serve warm.

Nutritional Facts (Per Serving): Calories: 500 | Fat: 5g | Carbs: 30g | Fiber: 9g | Sugars: 12g | Protein: 20g | Sodium: 350mg

Creamy Cauliflower and Broccoli Risotto

Prep: 10 minutes | Cook: 25 minutes | Serves: 1

Ingredients:

- 1/2 tbsp olive oil (7g)
- 1/4 cup Arborio rice (50g)
- 1/2 cup low-sodium vegetable broth (120ml)
- 1/4 cup chopped cauliflower (50g)
- 1/4 cup chopped broccoli (50g)
- 1/4 cup almond milk, unsweetened (60ml)
- 1 garlic clove, minced (3g)
- 1/4 tsp dried thyme (0.5g)
- Salt and pepper to taste

Instructions:

1. Heat olive oil in a pot over medium heat. Sauté garlic until fragrant, about 1 minute.

2. Add rice, stirring to coat, then add vegetable broth gradually, stirring frequently.

3. Add cauliflower and broccoli once the broth is halfway absorbed. Continue cooking, stirring, until rice is tender and creamy.

4. Stir in almond milk and thyme. Season with salt and pepper, and serve warm.

Nutritional Facts (Per Serving): Calories: 500 | Fat: 5g | Carbs: 30g | Fiber: 10g | Sugars: 13g | Protein: 20g | Sodium: 300mg

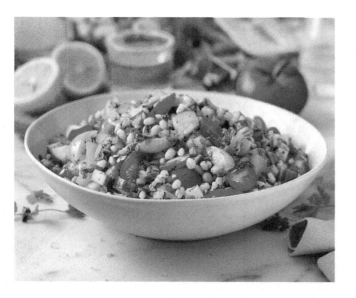

Lemon Herb Farro Pasta Salad

Prep: 15 minutes | Cook: 20 minutes | Serves: 1

Ingredients:

- 1/2 cup cooked farro (75g)
- 1/2 cup cherry tomatoes, halved (75g)
- 1/4 cup diced cucumber (40g)
- 1/4 cup diced bell pepper (40g)
- 1/2 tbsp olive oil (7g)
- Juice and zest of 1/2 lemon
- 1/4 tsp dried oregano (0.5g)
- 1/4 tsp dried basil (0.5g)
- Salt and pepper to taste

Instructions:

1. In a large bowl, combine the cooked farro, halved cherry tomatoes, diced cucumber, and diced bell pepper. Gently toss the ingredients together.
2. In a small bowl, whisk together the olive oil, lemon juice, lemon zest, dried oregano, dried basil, salt, and pepper until the dressing is smooth and well combined.
3. Taste the dressing and adjust seasoning if needed, adding more salt, pepper, or lemon juice to your preference.
4. Pour the dressing over the salad mixture and toss gently to coat all the ingredients evenly.
5. Let the salad sit for a few minutes to allow the flavors to meld, then serve chilled or at room temperature.

Nutritional Facts (Per Serving): Calories: 500 | Fat: 5g | Carbs: 30g | Fiber: 9g | Sugars: 12g | Protein: 20g | Sodium: 350mg

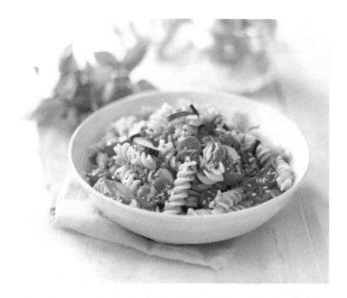

Zucchini and Tomato Basil Whole Grain Pasta

Prep: 10 minutes | Cook: 20 minutes | Serves: 1

Ingredients:

- 1/2 cup whole grain pasta (75g)
- 1/2 tbsp olive oil (7g)
- 1/2 cup diced zucchini (75g)
- 1/4 cup cherry tomatoes, halved (40g)
- 1 garlic clove, minced (3g)
- 1/4 tsp dried basil (0.5g)
- 1/4 tsp dried thyme (0.5g)
- Salt and pepper to taste

Instructions:

1. Cook the whole grain pasta according to the package directions. Once done, drain and set aside, reserving a small amount of pasta water.
2. Heat olive oil in a skillet over medium heat. Add the diced zucchini, halved cherry tomatoes, and minced garlic. Sauté, stirring occasionally, until the vegetables are tender, about 5 minutes.
3. Add the dried basil, dried thyme, salt, and pepper. Stir to combine and cook for another minute to enhance the flavors.
4. Add the cooked pasta to the skillet. Toss everything together, adding a small amount of reserved pasta water if the mixture is too dry.
5. Serve warm, adjusting seasoning to taste.

Nutritional Facts (Per Serving): Calories: 500 | Fat: 5g | Carbs: 30g | Fiber: 8g | Sugars: 13g | Protein: 20g | Sodium: 300mg

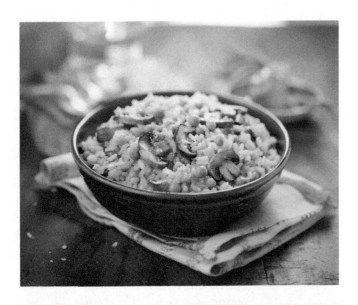

Mushroom and Pea Brown Rice Risotto

Prep: 10 minutes | Cook: 30 minutes | Serves: 1

Ingredients:

- 1/2 tbsp olive oil (7g)
- 1/4 cup diced onion (40g)
- 1 garlic clove, minced (3g)
- 1/2 cup sliced mushrooms (75g)
- 1/4 cup brown rice (50g)
- 1/2 cup low-sodium vegetable broth (120ml)
- 1/4 cup green peas (40g)
- 1 tbsp grated Parmesan cheese (5g)
- 1/4 tsp dried thyme (0.5g)
- Salt and pepper to taste

Instructions:

1. Heat olive oil in a pot over medium heat. Sauté onion, garlic, and mushrooms until softened, about 5 minutes.
2. Add brown rice and cook, stirring, for 1 minute.
3. Gradually add vegetable broth, stirring frequently until rice is tender, about 25 minutes.
4. Stir in green peas, Parmesan, thyme, salt, and pepper. Cook for 2-3 minutes until peas are heated through.
5. Adjust the seasoning if necessary, then serve warm.

Nutritional Facts (Per Serving): Calories: 500 | Fat: 5g | Carbs: 30g | Fiber: 9g | Sugars: 13g | Protein: 20g | Sodium: 350mg

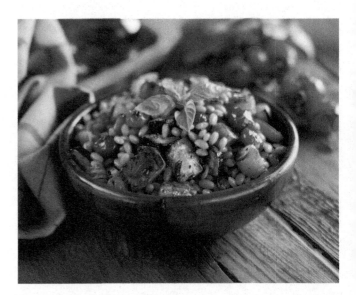

Roasted Vegetable and Barley Pasta

Prep: 15 minutes | Cook: 30 minutes | Serves: 1

Ingredients:

- 1/2 cup diced bell pepper (75g)
- 1/2 cup diced zucchini (75g)
- 1/2 cup cherry tomatoes, halved (75g)
- 1/2 tbsp olive oil (7g)
- 1/4 cup cooked barley (50g)
- 1/4 cup whole grain pasta (50g)
- 1/2 cup low-sodium vegetable broth (120ml)
- 1/4 tsp dried basil (0.5g)
- 1/4 tsp dried oregano (0.5g)
- Salt and pepper to taste

Instructions:

1. Preheat oven to 400°F (200°C). Toss bell pepper, zucchini, and cherry tomatoes with olive oil, salt, and pepper. Roast for 20 minutes.
2. Cook pasta according to package instructions. Drain and set aside.
3. In a pot, combine roasted vegetables, cooked barley, pasta, vegetable broth, basil, and oregano. Stir and heat through.
4. Season with additional salt and pepper to taste, and serve warm.

Nutritional Facts (Per Serving): Calories: 500 | Fat: 5g | Carbs: 30g | Fiber: 10g | Sugars: 12g | Protein: 20g | Sodium: 300mg

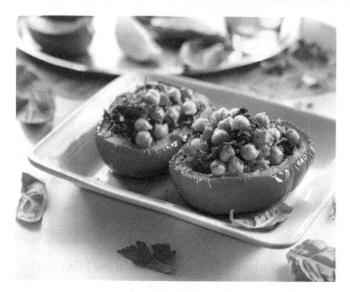

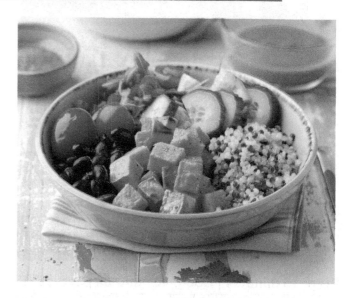

Chickpea and Spinach Stuffed Peppers

Prep: 15 minutes | Cook: 25 minutes | Serves: 1

Ingredients:

- 1 large bell pepper, halved and seeded (150g)
- 1/2 tbsp olive oil (7g)
- 1/4 cup canned chickpeas, rinsed (40g)
- 1/2 cup fresh spinach (15g)
- 1/4 cup diced tomatoes (60g)
- 1 garlic clove, minced (3g)
- 1/4 tsp dried oregano (0.5g)
- Salt and pepper to taste

Instructions:

1. Preheat oven to 400°F (200°C).
2. In a skillet, heat olive oil over medium heat. Sauté garlic, chickpeas, spinach, and tomatoes with oregano, salt, and pepper for 3-5 minutes until spinach is wilted.
3. Fill each pepper half with the chickpea-spinach mixture.
4. Place stuffed peppers in a baking dish, cover with foil, and bake for 20 minutes until peppers are tender. Serve warm.

Nutritional Facts (Per Serving): Calories: 500 | Fat: 5g | Carbs: 30g | Fiber: 9g | Sugars: 13g | Protein: 20 | Sodium: 350mg

Black Bean and Sweet Potato Buddha Bowl

Prep: 15 minutes | Cook: 25 minutes | Serves: 1

Ingredients:

- 1/2 cup diced sweet potato (75g)
- 1/2 tbsp olive oil (7g)
- 1/4 cup canned black beans, rinsed (40g)
- 1/4 cup cooked quinoa (50g)
- 1/4 cup diced cucumber (40g)
- 1/4 cup cherry tomatoes, halved (40g)
- 1 tbsp fresh lemon juice (15ml)
- 1/4 tsp ground cumin (0.5g)
- Salt and pepper to taste

Instructions:

1. Preheat oven to 400°F (200°C). Toss sweet potato with olive oil, salt, and pepper. Roast for 20 minutes until tender.
2. In a bowl, combine roasted sweet potato, black beans, quinoa, cucumber, and cherry tomatoes.
3. Drizzle with lemon juice, sprinkle with cumin, and season with salt and pepper. Serve warm.

Nutritional Facts (Per Serving): Calories: 500 | Fat: 5g | Carbs: 30g | Fiber: 10g | Sugars: 12g | Protein: 20g | Sodium: 300mg

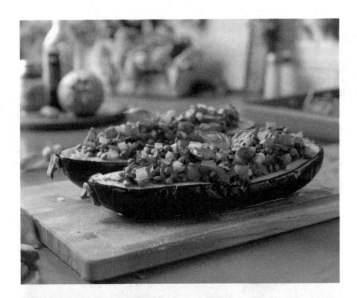

Lentil and Vegetable Stuffed Eggplant

Prep: 15 minutes | Cook: 40 minutes | Serves: 1

Ingredients:

- 1 medium eggplant (300g)
- 1/2 cup dry lentils (100g)
- 1 cup diced tomatoes (240g)
- 1/2 cup diced onion (80g)
- 1/2 cup diced bell pepper (75g)
- 2 cloves garlic, minced (6g)
- 1 tbsp olive oil (15g)
- 1 tsp dried oregano (1g)
- 1 tsp dried basil (1g)
- Salt and pepper to taste

Instructions:

1. Preheat oven to 375°F (190°C). Halve the eggplant lengthwise and scoop out the flesh, leaving a 1/4-inch (0.5 cm) thick shell. Chop the scooped-out flesh and set aside.
2. Cook lentils according to package instructions until tender. Drain and set aside.
3. In a skillet, heat olive oil over medium heat. Sauté onion, bell pepper, garlic, and chopped eggplant flesh for 5 minutes.
4. Add cooked lentils, diced tomatoes, oregano, basil, salt, and pepper. Cook for an additional 5 minutes.
5. Stuff the eggplant shells with the lentil mixture. Place them on a baking sheet.
6. Bake for 25-30 minutes until the eggplant shells are tender. Serve warm.

Nutritional Facts (Per Serving): Calories: 500 kcal | Fat: 5g | Carbs: 28g | Fiber: 9g | Sugars: 13g | Protein: 23g | Sodium: 350 mg

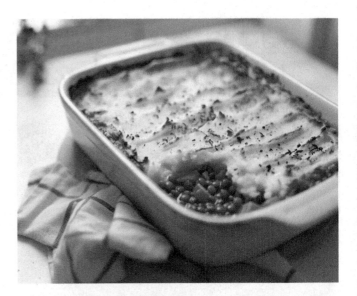

Vegetable and Lentil Shepherd's Pie

Prep: 20 minutes | Cook: 40 minutes | Serves: 1

Ingredients:

- 1/2 cup dry lentils (100g)
- 1 cup diced carrots (130g)
- 1 cup diced celery (100g)
- 1/2 cup diced onion (80g)
- 2 cloves garlic, minced (6g)
- 1 tbsp olive oil (15g)
- 1 cup low-sodium vegetable broth (240ml)
- 2 tbsp tomato paste (30g)
- 1 tsp dried thyme (1g)
- 1 cup mashed potatoes or cauliflower (200g)
- Salt and pepper to taste

Instructions:

1. Preheat oven to 375°F (190°C).
2. Cook lentils in vegetable broth until tender, about 20 minutes.
3. In a skillet, heat olive oil over medium heat. Sauté onion, carrots, celery, and garlic for 5 minutes until softened.
4. Add cooked lentils, tomato paste, thyme, salt, and pepper to the skillet. Stir well and cook for 5 more minutes.
5. Transfer the mixture to a baking dish. Spread mashed potatoes or cauliflower evenly over the top.
6. Bake for 20 minutes until the top is lightly browned. Serve hot.

Nutritional Facts (Per Serving): Calories: 500 kcal | Fat: 5g | Carbs: 28g | Fiber: 10g | Sugars: 12g | Protein: 24g | Sodium: 350 mg

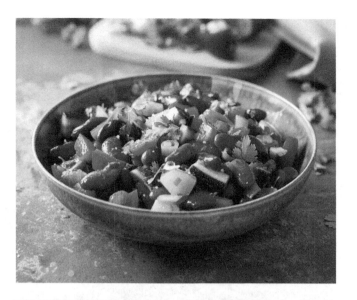

Spicy Kidney Bean and Veggie Stir-Fry

Prep: 10 minutes | Cook: 15 minutes | Serves: 1

Ingredients:

- 1/2 tbsp olive oil (7g)
- 1/2 cup canned kidney beans, rinsed (80g)
- 1/2 cup diced bell pepper (75g)
- 1/4 cup diced onion (40g)
- 1/4 cup sliced zucchini (40g)
- 1 garlic clove, minced (3g)
- 1/4 tsp ground cumin (0.5g)
- 1/4 tsp smoked paprika (0.5g)
- Salt and pepper to taste

Instructions:

1. Heat olive oil in a skillet over medium heat. Add the minced garlic, diced onion, bell pepper, and zucchini. Sauté, stirring occasionally, for about 5 minutes until the vegetables are softened.
2. Add the kidney beans to the skillet, along with the ground cumin, smoked paprika, salt, and pepper. Stir well to combine the ingredients and coat them evenly with the spices.
3. Continue cooking the mixture for another 5 minutes, stirring occasionally, until the beans are heated through and the flavors have melded.
4. Taste the stir-fry and adjust seasoning if needed by adding more salt, pepper, or spices.
5. Serve the stir-fry warm, either as a main dish or with a side of your choice.

Nutritional Facts (Per Serving): Calories: 500 | Fat: 5g | Carbs: 28g | Fiber: 9g | Sugars: 13g | Protein: 23g | Sodium: 350 mg

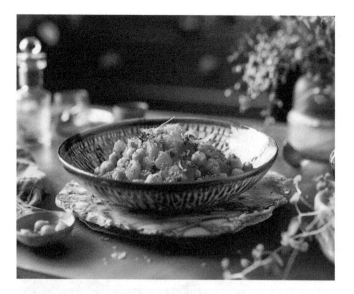

Butternut Squash and Chickpea Tagine

Prep: 15 minutes | Cook: 30 minutes | Serves: 1

Ingredients:

- 1/2 tbsp olive oil (7g)
- 1/2 cup diced butternut squash (75g)
- 1/2 cup canned chickpeas, rinsed (80g)
- 1/4 cup diced tomatoes (60g)
- 1/4 cup diced onion (40g)
- 1 garlic clove, minced (3g)
- 1/4 tsp ground cinnamon (0.5g)
- 1/4 tsp ground cumin (0.5g)
- 1/4 tsp ground coriander (0.5g)
- Salt and pepper to taste

Instructions:

1. Heat olive oil in a pot over medium heat. Add the minced garlic and diced onion. Sauté for about 5 minutes, stirring occasionally, until softened and fragrant.
2. Add the diced butternut squash, chickpeas, diced tomatoes, ground cinnamon, ground cumin, ground coriander, salt, and pepper. Stir everything together to combine.
3. If the mixture seems dry, add a splash of water to help cook the squash. Stir again and cover the pot.
4. Cook for 20-25 minutes, stirring occasionally, until the butternut squash is tender and the flavors have melded together. Serve warm.

Nutritional Facts (Per Serving): Calories: 500 | Fat: 5g | Carbs: 28g | Fiber: 10g | Sugars: 12g | Protein: 22g | Sodium: 300 mg

CHAPTER 11: LUNCHES: Lean Protein-Packed Lunches

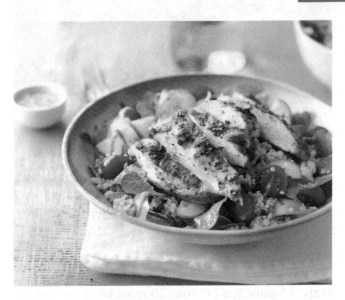

Grilled Chicken and Quinoa Salad

Prep: 10 minutes | Cook: 20 minutes | Serves: 1

Ingredients:

- 1 small chicken breast (120g)
- 1/2 tbsp olive oil (7g)
- Salt and pepper to taste
- 1/2 cup cooked quinoa (75g)
- 1/2 cup mixed salad greens (30g)
- 1/4 cup cherry tomatoes, halved (40g)
- 1/4 cup diced cucumber (40g)
- 1 tbsp lemon juice (15ml)

Instructions:

1. Preheat grill to medium heat. Season chicken breast with olive oil, salt, and pepper.
2. Grill chicken for 5-7 minutes per side, or until fully cooked. Let cool slightly, then slice.
3. In a bowl, combine quinoa, salad greens, cherry tomatoes, cucumber, and lemon juice. Toss gently.
4. Top the salad with grilled chicken slices and serve.

Nutritional Facts (Per Serving): Calories: 500 kcal | Fat: 5g | Carbs: 28g | Fiber: 9g | Sugars: 13g | Protein: 23g | Sodium: 350 mg

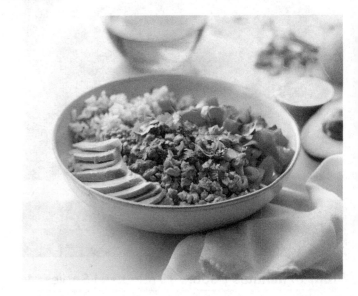

Turkey and Avocado Power Bowl

Prep: 10 minutes | Cook: 15 minutes | Serves: 1

Ingredients:

- 1/2 cup cooked ground turkey (120g)
- 1/2 tbsp olive oil (7g)
- Salt and pepper to taste
- 1/4 cup cooked brown rice (50g)
- 1/4 avocado, sliced (30g)
- 1/4 cup diced bell pepper (40g)
- 1/4 cup cherry tomatoes, halved (40g)
- 1 tbsp lime juice (15ml)

Instructions:

1. Heat olive oil in a skillet over medium heat. Add ground turkey, season with salt and pepper, and cook until browned, about 5-7 minutes.
2. In a bowl, layer brown rice, cooked turkey, avocado, bell pepper, and cherry tomatoes.
3. Drizzle with lime juice, season with additional salt and pepper if needed, and serve.

Nutritional Facts (Per Serving): Calories: 500 kcal | Fat: 5g | Carbs: 28g | Fiber: 8g | Sugars: 12g | Protein: 22g | Sodium: 300

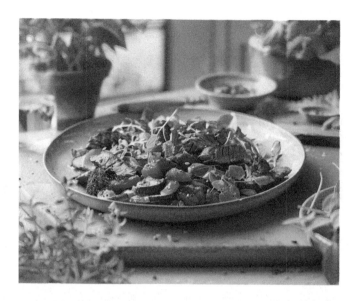

Lean Beef and Vegetable Stir-Fry

Prep: 10 minutes | Cook: 15 minutes | Serves: 1

Ingredients:

- 4 oz lean beef strips (120g)
- 1/2 tbsp olive oil (7g)
- 1/4 cup sliced bell pepper (40g)
- 1/4 cup sliced zucchini (40g)
- 1/4 cup broccoli florets (40g)
- 1 garlic clove, minced (3g)
- 1 tbsp low-sodium soy sauce (15ml)
- 1/4 tsp ground ginger (0.5g)
- Salt and pepper to taste

Instructions:

1. Heat olive oil in a skillet over medium-high heat. Add the minced garlic and beef strips. Stir-fry for 3-4 minutes, stirring frequently, until the beef is browned and cooked through.
2. Add the sliced bell pepper, zucchini, and broccoli florets to the skillet. Continue stir-frying for an additional 5 minutes until the vegetables are tender but still crisp.
3. Stir in the low-sodium soy sauce and ground ginger, ensuring the beef and vegetables are evenly coated. Season with salt and pepper to taste.
4. Cook for another 2 minutes, stirring occasionally, allowing the flavors to blend and the dish to heat through. Serve warm.

Nutritional Facts (Per Serving): Calories: 500 | Fat: 5g | Carbs: 28g | Fiber: 8g | Sugars: 12g | Protein: 23g | Sodium: 350 mg

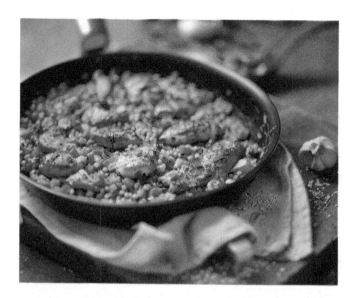

Herbed Chicken and Farro Pilaf

Prep: 10 minutes | Cook: 25 minutes | Serves: 1

Ingredients:

- 1 small chicken breast, diced (120g)
- 1/2 tbsp olive oil (7g)
- 1/2 cup cooked farro (75g)
- 1/4 cup diced carrots (40g)
- 1/4 cup diced celery (40g)
- 1 garlic clove, minced (3g)
- 1/4 tsp dried thyme (0.5g)
- 1/4 tsp dried rosemary (0.5g)
- Salt and pepper to taste

Instructions:

1. Heat olive oil in a skillet over medium heat. Add the minced garlic and diced chicken. Cook for about 5-6 minutes, stirring occasionally, until the chicken is browned and cooked through.
2. Add the diced carrots, celery, dried thyme, and dried rosemary to the skillet. Stir everything together and cook for about 5 minutes, until the vegetables are tender.
3. Stir in the cooked farro and season with salt and pepper to taste. Mix well to combine all the ingredients.
4. Cook for another 2 minutes, allowing the farro to heat through and absorb the flavors.
5. Taste and adjust seasoning if needed, then serve warm.

Nutritional Facts (Per Serving): Calories: 500 | Fat: 5g | Carbs: 28g | Fiber: 9g | Sugars: 13g | Protein: 24g | Sodium: 300 mg

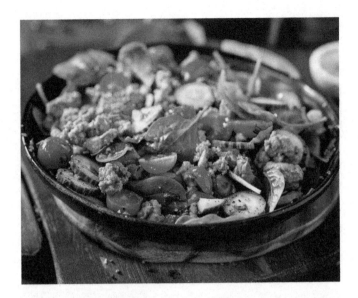

Lemon Garlic Turkey and Spinach Salad

Prep 10 minutes | Cook: 15 minutes | Serves: 1

Ingredients:

- 4 oz ground turkey (120g)
- 1/2 tbsp olive oil (7g)
- 1 garlic clove, minced (3g)
- Juice and zest of 1/2 lemon
- Salt and pepper to taste
- 2 cups fresh spinach (60g)
- 1/4 cup diced cucumber (40g)
- 1/4 cup cherry tomatoes, halved (40g)

Instructions:

1. Heat olive oil in a skillet over medium heat. Add the minced garlic and ground turkey. Season with salt and pepper. Cook for 5-6 minutes, breaking up the turkey with a spoon, until it's fully cooked and browned.

2. Add the lemon juice and zest to the turkey, stirring to evenly coat. Cook for an additional 1-2 minutes, allowing the flavors to blend.

3. In a separate bowl, combine the fresh spinach, diced cucumber, and halved cherry tomatoes. Toss together lightly to mix the vegetables.

4. Top the salad with the cooked turkey mixture, ensuring it's evenly distributed over the vegetables.

Nutritional Facts (Per Serving): Calories: 500 | Fat: 5g | Carbs: 30g | Fiber: 9g | Sugars: 13g | Protein: 22g | Sodium: 350 mg

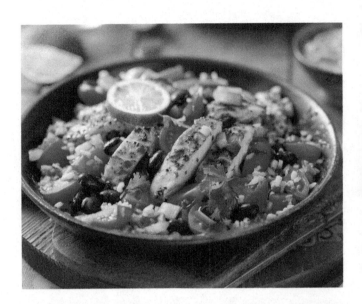

Chicken and Black Bean Fiesta Bowl

Prep: 10 minutes | Cook: 15 minutes | Serves: 1

Ingredients:

- 1 small chicken breast, diced (120g)
- 1/2 tbsp olive oil (7g)
- Salt and pepper to taste
- 1/4 cup canned black beans, rinsed (40g)
- 1/4 cup cooked brown rice (50g)
- 1/4 cup diced bell pepper (40g)
- 1/4 cup cherry tomatoes, halved (40g)
- 1 tbsp lime juice (15ml)

Instructions:

1. Heat olive oil in a skillet over medium heat. Season diced chicken with salt and pepper, then cook for 5-7 minutes, stirring occasionally, until the chicken is fully cooked and browned.

2. While the chicken is cooking, prepare the other ingredients. In a bowl, combine black beans, cooked brown rice, diced bell pepper, and halved cherry tomatoes.

3. Once the chicken is cooked, remove from heat and add it to the bowl with the other ingredients.

4. Gently toss everything together to combine evenly.

5. Drizzle with lime juice and stir to coat the ingredients well. Serve warm and enjoy!

Nutritional Facts (Per Serving): Calories: 500 | Fat: 5g | Carbs: 30g | Fiber: 10g | Sugars: 12g | Protein: 23g | Sodium: 300 mg

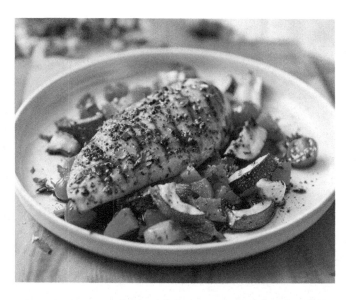

Balsamic Chicken and Roasted Veggies

Prep: 10 minutes | Cook: 20 minutes | Serves: 1

Ingredients:

- 1 small chicken breast (120g)
- 1 tbsp balsamic vinegar (15ml)
- 1/2 tbsp olive oil (7g)
- Salt and pepper to taste
- 1/4 cup diced zucchini (40g)
- 1/4 cup diced bell pepper (40g)
- 1/4 cup cherry tomatoes, halved (40g)
- 1/4 cup sliced carrots (40g)

Instructions:

1. Preheat oven to 400°F (200°C). In a bowl, toss chicken with balsamic vinegar, olive oil, salt, and pepper to coat evenly.
2. Arrange chicken and diced vegetables (zucchini, bell pepper, cherry tomatoes, and carrots) on a baking sheet, ensuring they are spread out in a single layer.
3. Roast for 20 minutes, or until chicken is cooked through and vegetables are tender.
4. Check the chicken's internal temperature to ensure it's fully cooked (165°F or 75°C).
5. Serve warm, garnishing with any additional balsamic vinegar if desired.

Nutritional Facts (Per Serving): Calories: 500 | Fat: 5g | Carbs: 29g | Fiber: 9g | Sugars: 13g | Protein: 22g | Sodium: 350 mg

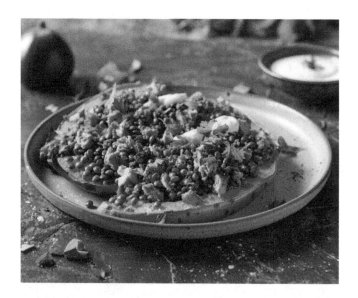

Turkey and Lentil Stuffed Sweet Potatoes

Prep: 10 minutes | Cook: 25 minutes | Serves: 1

Ingredients:

- 1 medium sweet potato (150g)
- 1/4 cup cooked ground turkey (60g)
- 1/4 cup cooked lentils (50g)
- 1/2 tbsp olive oil (7g)
- 1 garlic clove, minced (3g)
- 1/4 tsp ground cumin (0.5g)
- Salt and pepper to taste
- 1 tbsp Greek yogurt (15g) for topping

Instructions:

1. Preheat oven to 400°F (200°C). Pierce sweet potato with a fork and bake for 25 minutes, or until tender.
2. In a skillet, heat olive oil over medium heat. Add garlic, turkey, and lentils. Season with cumin, salt, and pepper. Cook for 5 minutes, stirring occasionally.
3. Slice baked sweet potato open and stuff with turkey-lentil mixture. Top with a dollop of Greek yogurt.
4. Serve immediately and enjoy!

Nutritional Facts (Per Serving): Calories: 500 | Fat: 5g | Carbs: 29g | Fiber: 10g | Sugars: 12g | Protein: 23g | Sodium: 300 mg

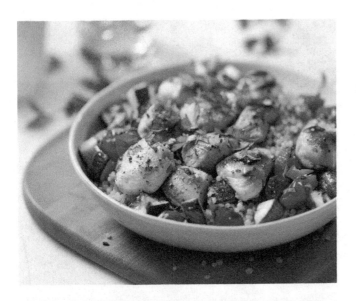

Chicken and Vegetable Medley Quinoa

Prep: 10 minutes | Cook: 20 minutes | Serves: 1

Ingredients:

- 1 small chicken breast, diced (120g)
- 1/2 tbsp olive oil (7g)
- Salt and pepper to taste
- 1/2 cup cooked quinoa (75g)
- 1/4 cup diced zucchini (40g)
- 1/4 cup diced bell pepper (40g)
- 1/4 cup cherry tomatoes, halved (40g)
- 1 tbsp fresh parsley, chopped (4g)

Instructions:

1. Preheat the oven to 400°F (200°C). In a bowl, toss diced chicken with olive oil, salt, and pepper to coat evenly.

2. Dice the zucchini, bell pepper, and cherry tomatoes. Arrange the chicken and vegetables on a baking sheet in a single layer.

3. Roast for 20 minutes, stirring halfway through, until chicken is cooked through and vegetables are tender.

4. Serve the roasted chicken and vegetables over quinoa, garnished with chopped parsley. Optionally, drizzle with extra balsamic vinegar.

Nutritional Facts (Per Serving): Calories: 500 | Fat: 5g | Carbs: 30g | Fiber: 9g | Sugars: 13g | Protein: 23g | Sodium: 350 mg

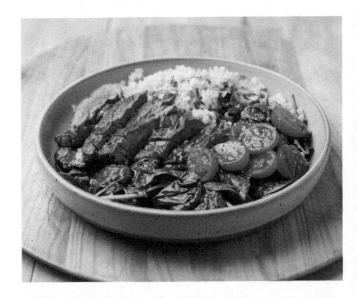

Lean Steak and Spinach Power Bowl

Prep: 10 minutes | Cook: 15 minutes | Serves: 1

Ingredients:

- 4 oz lean steak, sliced (120g)
- 1/2 tbsp olive oil (7g)
- Salt and pepper to taste
- 1/2 cup cooked brown rice (75g)
- 1 cup fresh spinach (30g)
- 1/4 cup cherry tomatoes, halved (40g)
- 1 tbsp balsamic vinegar (15ml)

Instructions:

1. Heat olive oil in a skillet over medium-high heat. Season the steak slices with salt and pepper. Cook for 3-4 minutes per side, or until the steak reaches your desired level of doneness. Once cooked, remove the steak from the skillet and set it aside to rest for a few minutes.

2. In a serving bowl, layer the cooked brown rice at the bottom. Add a layer of fresh spinach and cherry tomato halves on top. Slice the steak and arrange the slices over the vegetables.

3. Drizzle the assembled power bowl with balsamic vinegar and serve warm, mixing the ingredients together before eating.

Nutritional Facts (Per Serving): Calories: 500 | Fat: 5g | Carbs: 30g | Fiber: 8g | Sugars: 12g | Protein: 24g | Sodium: 300 mg

CHAPTER 12: SNACKS: Energizing Quick Bites

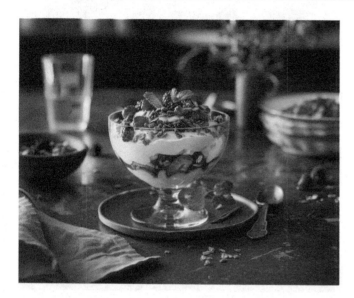

Greek Yogurt Parfait with Fresh Fruits

Prep: 10 minutes | Cook: None | Serves: 1

Ingredients:

- 1/2 cup Greek yogurt (125g)
- 1/4 cup mixed berries (blueberries, strawberries) (50g)
- 1 tbsp granola (10g)
- 1 tsp low carb sweetener (5g)
- 1/2 tsp vanilla extract (2.5g)

Instructions:

1. Mix Greek yogurt with vanilla extract and low carb sweetener in a small bowl.
2. Spoon half the yogurt mixture into a serving glass or bowl.
3. Layer half the mixed berries on top of the yogurt.
4. Add the remaining yogurt mixture and top with granola and the rest of the berries.
5. Serve immediately or chill for 5 minutes for flavors to blend.

Nutritional Facts (Per Serving): Calories: 220 | Fat: 5g | Sodium: 240mg | Carbs: 25g | Fiber: 4g | Sugars: 7g | Protein: 9g

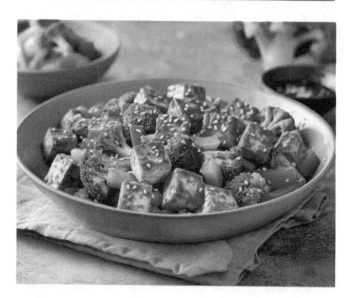

Spicy Tofu and Vegetable Bowl

Prep: 15 minutes | Cook: 10 minutes | Serves: 1

Ingredients:

- 1/2 block firm tofu, cubed (150g)
- 1/2 cup broccoli florets (50g)
- 1/4 cup sliced bell peppers (50g)
- 1 tbsp olive oil (15g)
- 1 tsp low sodium soy sauce (5g)
- 1/4 tsp chili flakes (1g)
- 1 tsp sesame seeds (5g)

Instructions:

1. Heat olive oil in a skillet over medium heat.
2. Add tofu cubes and sauté until golden brown, about 3-4 minutes.
3. Add broccoli and bell peppers to the skillet, cooking for another 4-5 minutes until tender-crisp.
4. Stir in soy sauce, chili flakes, and sesame seeds, tossing to coat evenly.
5. Serve hot in a bowl, garnished with extra sesame seeds if desired.

Nutritional Facts (Per Serving): Calories: 220 | Fat: 7g | Sodium: 290mg | Carbs: 15g | Fiber: 4g | Sugars: 6g | Protein: 10g

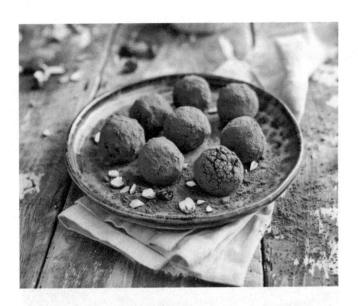

Almond & Date Energy Balls

Prep: 10 minutes | Cook: None | Serves: 1

Ingredients:

- 1/4 cup almonds (35g)
- 2 medjool dates, pitted (30g)
- 1 tsp low carb sweetener (5g)
- 1/2 tsp vanilla extract (2.5g)
- 1/2 tsp unsweetened cocoa powder (2.5g)

Instructions:

1. In a food processor, pulse the almonds until finely chopped.
2. Add dates, low carb sweetener, vanilla extract, and cocoa powder. Blend until the mixture forms a sticky dough.
3. Divide the mixture into small portions and roll into 4 bite-sized balls.
4. Place the energy balls on a plate or in a container.
5. Chill for 5 minutes before serving or store in the refrigerator for up to 5 days.

Nutritional Facts (Per Serving): Calories: 220 | Fat: 6g | Sodium: 230mg | Carbs: 24g | Fiber: 4g | Sugars: 7g | Protein: 8g

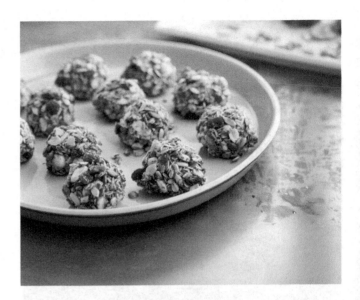

Trail Mix Power Clusters

Prep: 10 minutes | Cook: None | Serves: 1

Ingredients:

- 2 tbsp mixed nuts (almonds, walnuts) (20g)
- 1 tbsp sunflower seeds (10g)
- 1 tbsp dried cranberries (10g)
- 1 tsp low carb sweetener (5g)
- 1 tbsp almond butter (15g)

Instructions:

1. In a small bowl, combine the mixed nuts, sunflower seeds, and dried cranberries.
2. Add almond butter and low carb sweetener, mixing until the ingredients are fully coated.
3. Divide the mixture into clusters and shape them into small mounds.
4. Place the clusters on a plate lined with parchment paper.
5. Chill for 10 minutes before serving or store in an airtight container in the refrigerator.

Nutritional Facts (Per Serving): Calories: 220 | Fat: 7g | Sodium: 240mg | Carbs: 23g | Fiber: 5g | Sugars: 6g | Protein: 9g

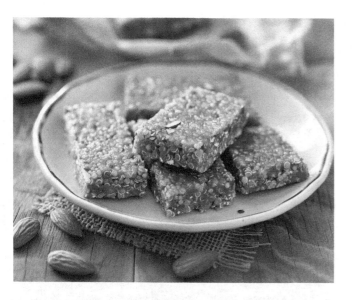

Nutty Quinoa Energy Bars

Prep: 15 minutes | Cook: 20 minutes | Serves: 1

Ingredients:

- 1/4 cup cooked quinoa (43g)
- 2 tbsp almond butter (30g)
- 1 tbsp chopped almonds (15g)
- 1 tbsp low carb sweetener (15g)
- 1/4 tsp cinnamon (0.5g)
- 1/4 tsp vanilla extract (1.25g)

Instructions:

1. Preheat the oven to 350°F (175°C) and line a small baking dish with parchment paper.
2. In a bowl, mix cooked quinoa, almond butter, chopped almonds, low carb sweetener, cinnamon, and vanilla extract until well combined.
3. Press the mixture evenly into the prepared baking dish.
4. Bake for 20 minutes, then let cool completely before slicing into bars.
5. Store in an airtight container in the refrigerator for up to 5 days.

Nutritional Facts (Per Serving): Calories: 220 | Fat: 6g | Sodium: 250mg | Carbs: 20g | Fiber: 5g | Sugars: 7g | Protein: 9g

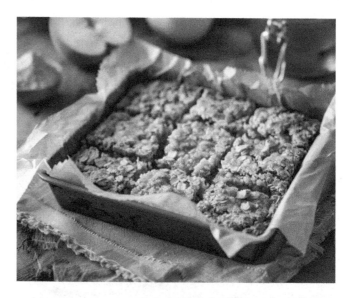

Apple Cinnamon Oat Bars

Prep: 10 minutes | Cook: 20 minutes | Serves: 1

Ingredients:

- 1/4 cup rolled oats (20g)
- 2 tbsp unsweetened applesauce (30g)
- 1 tbsp low carb sweetener (15g)
- 1/4 tsp ground cinnamon (0.5g)
- 1 tbsp chopped walnuts (15g)
- 1/4 tsp vanilla extract (1.25g)

Instructions:

1. Preheat the oven to 350°F (175°C) and line a small baking dish with parchment paper.
2. In a bowl, mix rolled oats, applesauce, low carb sweetener, ground cinnamon, walnuts, and vanilla extract until well combined.
3. Spread the mixture evenly into the prepared baking dish.
4. Bake for 20 minutes, then let cool completely before slicing into bars.
5. Store in an airtight container in the refrigerator for up to 5 days.

Nutritional Facts (Per Serving): Calories: 220 | Fat: 5g | Sodium: 240mg | Carbs: 25g | Fiber: 4g | Sugars: 6g | Protein: 8g

CHAPTER 13: SNACKS: Homemade Dips, Spreads, And Flavorful Low-Sodium Sauces

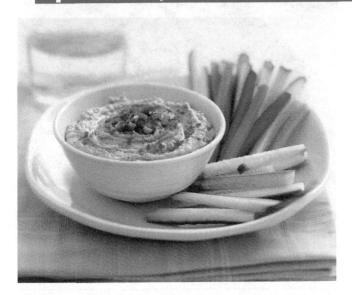

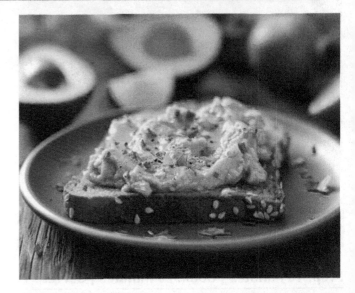

Roasted Red Pepper Hummus with Fresh Vegetable Sticks

Prep: 10 minutes | Cook: None | Serves: 1

Ingredients:

- 1/4 cup canned chickpeas, drained and rinsed (60g)
- 2 tbsp roasted red peppers (30g)
- 1 tsp olive oil (5g)
- 1/4 tsp ground cumin (0.5g)
- 1/2 tsp lemon juice (2.5g)
- 1/4 cup fresh vegetable sticks (carrots, celery, cucumber) (50g)

Instructions:

1. In a food processor, combine chickpeas, roasted red peppers, olive oil, cumin, and lemon juice.
2. Blend until smooth, adding a small amount of water if needed for desired consistency.
3. Transfer the hummus to a serving dish.
4. Arrange fresh vegetable sticks on a plate alongside the hummus.
5. Serve immediately or store the hummus in an airtight container in the refrigerator for up to 3 days.

Nutritional Facts (Per Serving): Calories: 220 | Fat: 6g | Sodium: 280mg | Carbs: 20g | Fiber: 5g | Sugars: 6g | Protein: 8g

Avocado Cilantro Lime Spread with Whole-Grain Toast

Prep: 10 minutes | Cook: None | Serves: 1

Ingredients:

- 1/4 avocado, mashed (30g)
- 1/2 tsp lime juice (2.5g)
- 1 tsp chopped fresh cilantro (1g)
- 1 slice whole-grain toast (30g)
- 1/4 tsp low carb sweetener (optional) (1g)

Instructions:

1. In a small bowl, mash the avocado with lime juice and cilantro until smooth.
2. Toast the slice of whole-grain bread to your preference.
3. Spread the avocado mixture evenly over the toast.
4. Sprinkle with a pinch of low carb sweetener if desired.
5. Serve immediately as a light snack or breakfast option.

Nutritional Facts (Per Serving): Calories: 220 | Fat: 7g | Sodium: 230mg | Carbs: 22g | Fiber: 5g | Sugars: 6g | Protein: 9g

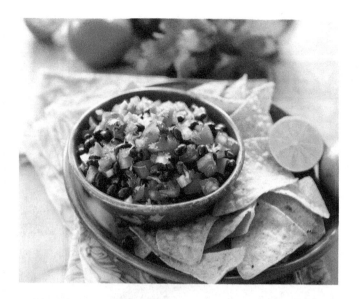

Spicy Black Bean Salsa with Whole-Grain Tortilla Chips

Prep: 10 minutes | Cook: None | Serves: 1

Ingredients:

- 1/4 cup canned black beans, rinsed and drained (60g)
- 2 tbsp diced tomatoes (30g)
- 1 tbsp diced red onion (15g)
- 1 tsp chopped fresh cilantro (1g)
- 1/2 tsp lime juice (2.5g)
- 1/4 tsp ground cumin (0.5g)
- 1/4 tsp chili powder (0.5g)
- 5 whole-grain tortilla chips (30g)

Instructions:

1. In a small bowl, combine black beans, diced tomatoes, red onion, and cilantro.
2. Add lime juice, cumin, and chili powder, mixing until evenly coated.
3. Serve the salsa in a small bowl alongside the tortilla chips.
4. Garnish with additional cilantro if desired.
5. Enjoy immediately as a light snack or appetizer.

Nutritional Facts (Per Serving): Calories: 220 | Fat: 6g | Sodium: 290mg | Carbs: 26g | Fiber: 5g | Sugars: 6g | Protein: 8g

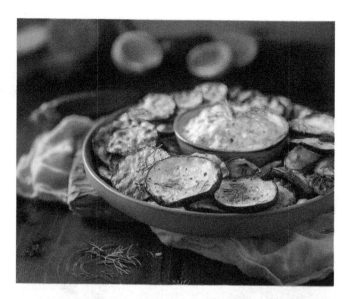

Zesty Lemon Herb Tzatziki with Baked Zucchini Chips

Prep: 10 minutes | Cook: 15 minutes | Serves: 1

Ingredients:

- 1/4 cup plain Greek yogurt (60g)
- 1/2 tsp lemon juice (2.5g)
- 1/4 tsp lemon zest (0.5g)
- 1/2 tsp chopped fresh dill (1g)
- 1/2 tsp minced garlic (2.5g)
- 1/4 tsp low carb sweetener (1g)
- 1 small zucchini, sliced into thin rounds (100g)
- 1 tsp olive oil (5g)

Instructions:

1. Preheat the oven to 375°F (190°C) and line a baking sheet with parchment paper.
2. Toss zucchini slices with olive oil and arrange them in a single layer on the prepared baking sheet. Bake for 12-15 minutes until crisp.
3. In a small bowl, mix Greek yogurt, lemon juice, lemon zest, dill, garlic, and low carb sweetener.
4. Serve the tzatziki dip in a bowl with the baked zucchini chips on the side.
5. Enjoy as a refreshing and healthy snack or appetizer.

Nutritional Facts (Per Serving): Calories: 220 | Fat: 7g | Sodium: 270mg | Carbs: 18g | Fiber: 4g | Sugars: 7g | Protein: 9g

CHAPTER 14: DESSERTS: Delectable Natural Desserts That Satisfy Your Sweet Tooth

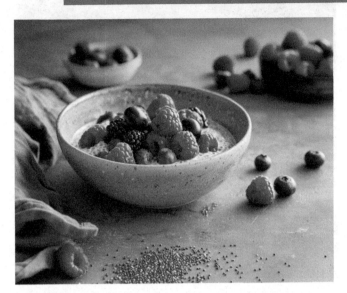

Chia Seed Pudding with Berries

Prep: 10 minutes | Cook: None (Chill: 4 hours) | Serves: 1

Ingredients:

- 2 tbsp chia seeds (30g)
- 1/2 cup unsweetened almond milk (120ml)
- 1 tsp low carb sweetener (5g)
- 1/4 tsp vanilla extract (1.25g)
- 1/4 cup mixed berries (blueberries, raspberries) (50g)

Instructions:

1. In a small bowl or jar, mix chia seeds, almond milk, low carb sweetener, and vanilla extract.
2. Stir well to prevent clumping and let it sit for 5 minutes. Stir again.
3. Cover and refrigerate for at least 4 hours or overnight until thickened.
4. Before serving, give the pudding a good stir and top with mixed berries.
5. Serve immediately or keep refrigerated for up to 3 days.

Nutritional Facts (Per Serving): Calories: 220 | Fat: 6g | Sodium: 240mg | Carbs: 22g | Fiber: 5g | Sugars: 7g | Protein: 8g

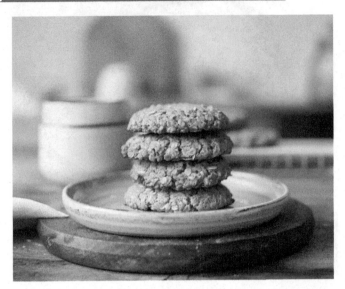

Banana Oatmeal Cookies

Prep: 10 minutes | Cook: 15 minutes | Serves: 1

Ingredients:

- 1/4 cup mashed ripe banana (60g)
- 2 tbsp rolled oats (15g)
- 1 tbsp almond flour (15g)
- 1 tsp low carb sweetener (5g)
- 1/4 tsp ground cinnamon (0.5g)
- 1 tbsp chopped walnuts (15g)

Instructions:

1. Preheat the oven to 350°F (175°C) and line a baking sheet with parchment paper.
2. In a small bowl, mix mashed banana, rolled oats, almond flour, low carb sweetener, and ground cinnamon until combined.
3. Fold in the chopped walnuts.
4. Drop spoonfuls of the mixture onto the prepared baking sheet and flatten slightly.
5. Bake for 12-15 minutes until golden brown. Let cool before serving.

Nutritional Facts (Per Serving): Calories: 220 | Fat: 7g | Sodium: 230mg | Carbs: 28g | Fiber: 4g | Sugars: 7g | Protein: 8g

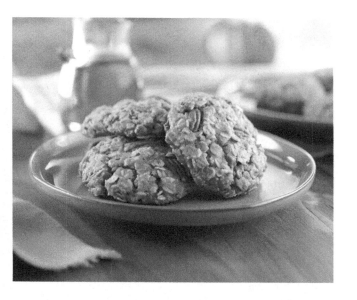

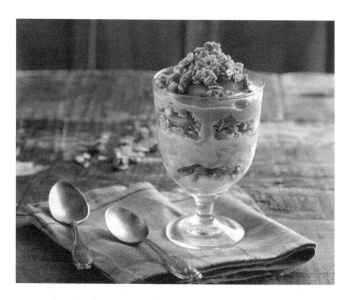

Pumpkin Spice Oatmeal Cookies

Prep: 10 minutes | Cook: 15 minutes | Serves: 1

Ingredients:

- 1/4 cup rolled oats (20g)
- 1 tbsp almond flour (15g)
- 1 tbsp pumpkin puree (15g)
- 1 tsp low carb sweetener (5g)
- 1/4 tsp pumpkin spice mix (0.5g)
- 1 tbsp chopped pecans (10g)

Instructions:

1. Preheat the oven to 350°F (175°C) and line a baking sheet with parchment paper.
2. In a small bowl, mix rolled oats, almond flour, pumpkin puree, low carb sweetener, and pumpkin spice mix until combined.
3. Fold in the chopped pecans.
4. Drop spoonfuls of the dough onto the prepared baking sheet and flatten slightly.
5. Bake for 12-15 minutes until golden brown. Let cool before serving.

Nutritional Facts (Per Serving): Calories: 220 | Fat: 6g | Sodium: 230mg | Carbs: 27g | Fiber: 5g | Sugars: 7g | Protein: 8g

Pumpkin Spice Yogurt Parfait

Prep: 10 minutes | Cook: None | Serves: 1

Ingredients:

- 1/2 cup plain Greek yogurt (125g)
- 2 tbsp pumpkin puree (30g)
- 1 tsp low carb sweetener (5g)
- 1/4 tsp pumpkin spice mix (0.5g)
- 1 tbsp granola (10g)

Instructions:

1. In a small bowl, mix Greek yogurt, pumpkin puree, low carb sweetener, and pumpkin spice mix until smooth.
2. Spoon half the yogurt mixture into a serving glass or bowl.
3. Add a layer of granola on top.
4. Repeat with the remaining yogurt mixture and finish with a sprinkle of granola.
5. Serve immediately or chill for 5 minutes before serving.

Nutritional Facts (Per Serving): Calories: 220 | Fat: 5g | Sodium: 240mg | Carbs: 22g | Fiber: 4g | Sugars: 7g | Protein: 9g

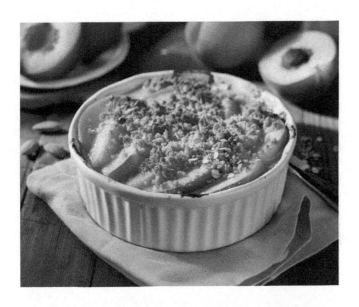

Peach and Almond Crisp

Prep: 10 minutes | Cook: 20 minutes | Serves: 1

Ingredients:

- 1/2 cup sliced peaches (100g)
- 1 tbsp almond flour (15g)
- 1 tbsp rolled oats (10g)
- 1 tsp low carb sweetener (5g)
- 1/4 tsp cinnamon (0.5g)
- 1 tsp chopped almonds (5g)

Instructions:

1. Preheat the oven to 350°F (175°C) and grease a small ramekin with cooking spray.
2. Arrange the peach slices in the ramekin.
3. In a small bowl, mix almond flour, rolled oats, low carb sweetener, cinnamon, and chopped almonds.
4. Sprinkle the mixture evenly over the peaches.
5. Bake for 20 minutes or until the top is golden brown and the peaches are tender. Let cool slightly before serving.

Nutritional Facts (Per Serving): Calories: 220 | Fat: 6g | Sodium: 230mg | Carbs: 25g | Fiber: 5g | Sugars: 7g | Protein: 8g

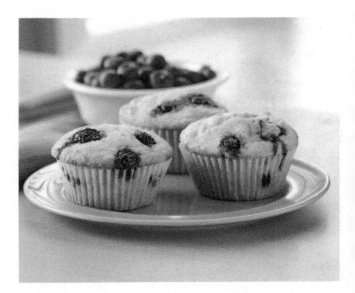

Blueberry Almond Flour Muffins

Prep: 10 minutes | Cook: 20 minutes | Serves: 1

Ingredients:

- 2 tbsp almond flour (30g)
- 1 tbsp plain Greek yogurt (15g)
- 1 tbsp blueberries (10g)
- 1 tsp low carb sweetener (5g)
- 1/4 tsp baking powder (1g)
- 1/4 tsp vanilla extract (1.25g)

Instructions:

1. Preheat the oven to 350°F (175°C) and line a muffin tin with a paper liner.
2. In a small bowl, mix almond flour, Greek yogurt, low carb sweetener, baking powder, and vanilla extract until smooth.
3. Fold in the blueberries.
4. Pour the batter into the prepared muffin liner.
5. Bake for 18-20 minutes or until a toothpick inserted in the center comes out clean. Let cool before serving.

Nutritional Facts (Per Serving): Calories: 220 | Fat: 7g | Sodium: 240mg | Carbs: 22g | Fiber: 4g | Sugars: 6g | Protein: 9g

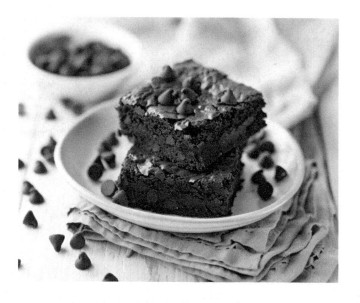

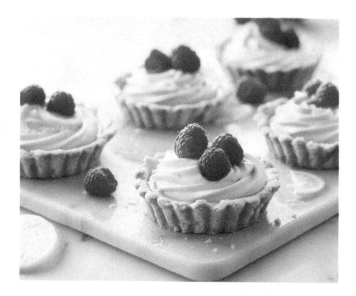

Dark Chocolate Avocado Brownies

Prep: 10 minutes | Cook: 20 minutes | Serves: 1

Ingredients:

- 2 tbsp mashed avocado (30g)
- 1 tbsp almond flour (15g)
- 1 tbsp unsweetened cocoa powder (10g)
- 1 tsp low carb sweetener (5g)
- 1 tbsp dark chocolate chips (15g)
- 1/4 tsp baking powder (1g)
- 1/4 tsp vanilla extract (1.25g)

Instructions:

1. Preheat the oven to 350°F (175°C) and grease a small ramekin or baking dish.
2. In a bowl, mix mashed avocado, almond flour, cocoa powder, low carb sweetener, baking powder, and vanilla extract until smooth.
3. Fold in dark chocolate chips.
4. Pour the mixture into the prepared ramekin and spread evenly.
5. Bake for 18-20 minutes or until a toothpick inserted in the center comes out clean. Let cool before serving.

Nutritional Facts (Per Serving): Calories: 220 | Fat: 7g | Sodium: 240mg | Carbs: 22g | Fiber: 5g | Sugars: 6g | Protein: 8g

Raspberry Lemon Tartlets

Prep: 15 minutes | Cook: 10 minutes | Serves: 1

Ingredients:

- 2 tbsp almond flour (30g)
- 1/2 tsp lemon juice (2.5g)
- 1 tsp low carb sweetener (5g)
- 1 tbsp Greek yogurt (15g)
- 2 fresh raspberries (10g)
- 1/4 tsp lemon zest (0.5g)

Instructions:

1. Preheat the oven to 350°F (175°C) and grease a mini tartlet mold or muffin tin.
2. In a small bowl, mix almond flour, lemon juice, and low carb sweetener to form a dough.
3. Press the dough into the mold to form a tart shell. Bake for 8-10 minutes until lightly golden. Let cool.
4. Fill the cooled tart shell with Greek yogurt and top with fresh raspberries and lemon zest.
5. Serve immediately or refrigerate for up to 1 day.

Nutritional Facts (Per Serving): Calories: 220 | Fat: 6g | Sodium: 230mg | Carbs: 20g | Fiber: 4g | Sugars: 7g | Protein: 9g

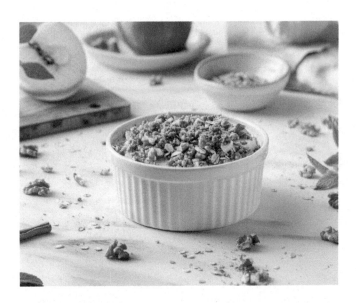

Apple Walnut Crumble

Prep: 10 minutes | Cook: 20 minutes | Serves: 1

Ingredients:

- 1/2 cup diced apple (75g)
- 1 tbsp rolled oats (10g)
- 1 tbsp almond flour (15g)
- 1 tsp low carb sweetener (5g)
- 1/4 tsp cinnamon (0.5g)
- 1 tbsp chopped walnuts (10g)

Instructions:

1. Preheat the oven to 350°F (175°C) and grease a small ramekin with cooking spray.
2. Place the diced apple in the ramekin and sprinkle with cinnamon.
3. In a small bowl, mix rolled oats, almond flour, low carb sweetener, and chopped walnuts.
4. Sprinkle the oat mixture evenly over the apples.
5. Bake for 20 minutes or until the top is golden brown and the apples are tender. Let cool slightly before serving.

Nutritional Facts (Per Serving): Calories: 220 | Fat: 6g | Sodium: 230mg | Carbs: 26g | Fiber: 5g | Sugars: 7g | Protein: 8g

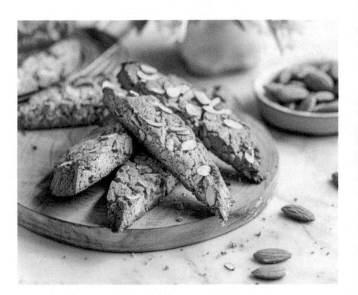

Orange Almond Whole Grain Biscotti

Prep: 15 minutes | Cook: 25 minutes | Serves: 1

Ingredients:

- 2 tbsp whole wheat flour (30g)
- 1 tbsp almond flour (15g)
- 1 tsp orange zest (5g)
- 1 tsp low carb sweetener (5g)
- 1/4 tsp baking powder (1g)
- 1 tbsp chopped almonds (10g)
- 1 tsp orange juice (5g)

Instructions:

1. Preheat the oven to 350°F (175°C) and line a baking sheet with parchment paper.
2. In a small bowl, mix whole wheat flour, almond flour, orange zest, low carb sweetener, and baking powder.
3. Add orange juice and stir until a dough forms. Fold in the chopped almonds.
4. Shape the dough into a small log and place it on the prepared baking sheet. Bake for 15 minutes.
5. Remove from the oven, slice into biscotti, and bake for another 10 minutes until crisp. Let cool before serving.

Nutritional Facts (Per Serving): Calories: 220 | Fat: 7g | Sodium: 240mg | Carbs: 24g | Fiber: 4g | Sugars: 6g | Protein: 9g

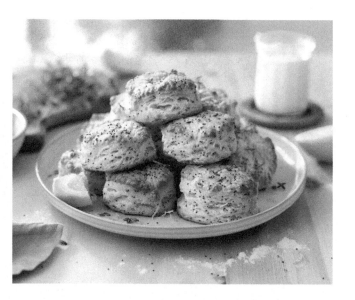

Lemon Poppy Seed Whole Wheat Scones

Prep: 15 minutes | Cook: 20 minutes | Serves: 1

Ingredients:

- 2 tbsp whole wheat flour (30g)
- 1 tsp poppy seeds (5g)
- 1 tsp low carb sweetener (5g)
- 1/4 tsp baking powder (1g)
- 1 tsp lemon zest (5g)
- 1 tbsp unsweetened almond milk (15ml)
- 1 tsp olive oil (5g)

Instructions:

1. Preheat the oven to 350°F (175°C) and line a baking sheet with parchment paper.
2. In a bowl, mix whole wheat flour, poppy seeds, low carb sweetener, baking powder, and lemon zest.
3. Add almond milk and olive oil, stirring until a dough forms.
4. Shape the dough into a small round and place it on the baking sheet.
5. Bake for 18-20 minutes until golden brown. Let cool before serving.

Nutritional Facts (Per Serving): Calories: 220 | Fat: 6g | Sodium: 230mg | Carbs: 25g | Fiber: 5g | Sugars: 6g | Protein: 8g

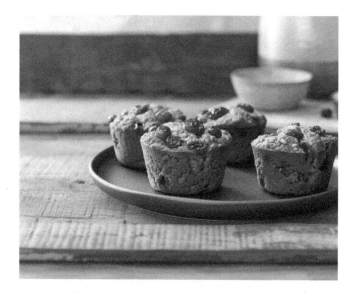

Cranberry Orange Whole Wheat Muffins

Prep: 15 minutes | Cook: 20 minutes | Serves: 1

Ingredients:

- 2 tbsp whole wheat flour (30g)
- 1 tbsp unsweetened dried cranberries (10g)
- 1 tsp orange zest (5g)
- 1 tsp low carb sweetener (5g)
- 1/4 tsp baking powder (1g)
- 1 tbsp unsweetened almond milk (15ml)
- 1 tsp olive oil (5g)

Instructions:

1. Preheat the oven to 350°F (175°C) and line a muffin tin with a paper liner.
2. In a bowl, mix whole wheat flour, cranberries, orange zest, low carb sweetener, and baking powder.
3. Add almond milk and olive oil, stirring until a batter forms.
4. Pour the batter into the prepared muffin liner.
5. Bake for 18-20 minutes until a toothpick inserted in the center comes out clean. Let cool before serving.

Nutritional Facts (Per Serving): Calories: 220 | Fat: 6g | Sodium: 240mg | Carbs: 24g | Fiber: 4g | Sugars: 7g | Protein: 8g

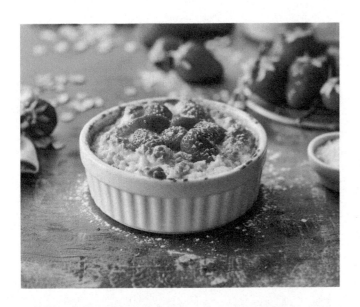

Strawberry Oatmeal Shortcake

Prep: 10 minutes | Cook: 15 minutes | Serves: 1

Ingredients:

- 1/4 cup rolled oats (20g)
- 1 tbsp almond flour (15g)
- 1 tsp low carb sweetener (5g)
- 1 tbsp plain Greek yogurt (15g)
- 1/4 cup diced strawberries (50g)
- 1/4 tsp vanilla extract (1.25g)

Instructions:

1. Preheat the oven to 350°F (175°C) and grease a small ramekin or baking dish.
2. In a bowl, mix rolled oats, almond flour, low carb sweetener, Greek yogurt, and vanilla extract until combined.
3. Pour the mixture into the ramekin and spread evenly.
4. Top with diced strawberries and bake for 15 minutes or until the oats are set.
5. Let cool slightly before serving.

Nutritional Facts (Per Serving): Calories: 220 | Fat: 6g | Sodium: 230mg | Carbs: 25g | Fiber: 5g | Sugars: 7g | Protein: 8g

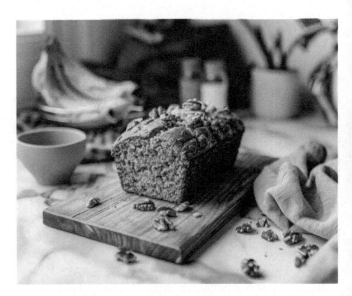

Banana Walnut Whole Grain Bread

Prep: 15 minutes | Cook: 25 minutes | Serves: 1

Ingredients:

- 2 tbsp whole wheat flour (30g)
- 1 tbsp mashed banana (15g)
- 1 tsp low carb sweetener (5g)
- 1/4 tsp baking powder (1g)
- 1 tbsp chopped walnuts (10g)
- 1 tbsp unsweetened almond milk (15ml)

Instructions:

1. Preheat the oven to 350°F (175°C) and line a small loaf pan with parchment paper.
2. In a bowl, mix whole wheat flour, mashed banana, low carb sweetener, baking powder, and almond milk until smooth.
3. Fold in chopped walnuts.
4. Pour the batter into the prepared loaf pan and smooth the top.
5. Bake for 25 minutes or until a toothpick inserted into the center comes out clean. Let cool before slicing.

Nutritional Facts (Per Serving): Calories: 220 | Fat: 7g | Sodium: 240mg | Carbs: 24g | Fiber: 5g | Sugars: 7g | Protein: 8g

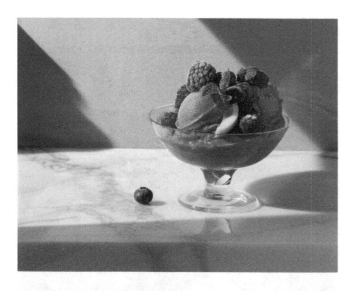

Mixed Berry Sorbet

Prep: 10 minutes | Cook: None (Freeze: 2 hours) | Serves: 1

Ingredients:

- 1/2 cup mixed berries (blueberries, raspberries, strawberries) (75g)
- 1 tbsp lemon juice (15ml)
- 1 tsp low carb sweetener (5g)
- 2 tbsp unsweetened almond milk (30ml)

Instructions:

1. In a blender, combine mixed berries, lemon juice, low carb sweetener, and almond milk.
2. Blend until smooth and creamy.
3. Transfer the mixture to a shallow, freezer-safe container.
4. Freeze for 2 hours, stirring every 30 minutes to prevent large ice crystals.
5. Scoop and serve immediately or store in the freezer for up to 2 days.

Nutritional Facts (Per Serving): Calories: 220 | Fat: 5g | Sodium: 240mg | Carbs: 25g | Fiber: 5g | Sugars: 7g | Protein: 8g

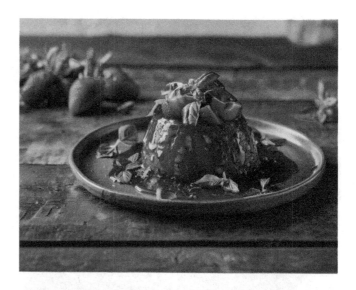

Strawberry Basil Gelée

Prep: 15 minutes | Cook: 5 minutes (Chill: 2 hours) | Serves: 1

Ingredients:

- 1/2 cup fresh strawberries, sliced (75g)
- 1 tbsp fresh basil, chopped (5g)
- 1/2 tsp lemon zest (2.5g)
- 1 tsp low carb sweetener (5g)
- 1/2 tsp unflavored gelatin powder (2.5g)
- 1 tbsp water (15ml)

Instructions:

1. In a small saucepan, combine strawberries, basil, lemon zest, and low carb sweetener. Cook over medium heat for 3 minutes until soft.
2. Dissolve gelatin in water and stir into the strawberry mixture. Remove from heat.
3. Pour the mixture into a small ramekin or mold.
4. Chill in the refrigerator for at least 2 hours until set.
5. Serve as is or unmold onto a plate.

Nutritional Facts (Per Serving): Calories: 220 | Fat: 5g | Sodium: 230mg | Carbs: 24g | Fiber: 5g | Sugars: 7g | Protein: 8g

CHAPTER 15: DINNER: Crisp And Nourishing Evening Salads

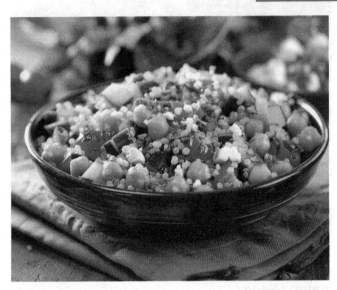

Mediterranean Chickpea and Quinoa Salad

Prep: 15 minutes | Cook: 15 minutes | Serves: 2

Ingredients:

- 1/2 cup cooked quinoa (85g)
- 1/2 cup cooked chickpeas (85g)
- 1/2 cup diced cucumber (75g)
- 1/2 cup halved cherry tomatoes (75g)
- 1/4 cup crumbled feta cheese (30g)
- 2 tbsp olive oil (30ml)
- 1 tbsp fresh lemon juice (15ml)
- 1 tsp dried oregano (2g)
- 1/4 tsp salt (1g)
- 1/4 tsp black pepper (1g)
- 2 tbsp chopped fresh parsley (8g)

Instructions:

1. In a large bowl, combine quinoa, chickpeas, cucumber, cherry tomatoes, and feta cheese.
2. In a small bowl, whisk together olive oil, lemon juice, oregano, salt, and black pepper to make the dressing.
3. Pour the dressing over the salad ingredients and toss gently to coat.
4. Add the chopped parsley and toss again to combine. Serve immediately.

Nutritional Facts (Per Serving): Calories: 380 | Fat: 14g | Carbs: 47g | Fiber: 8g | Sugars: 4g | Protein: 14g | Sodium: 400mg

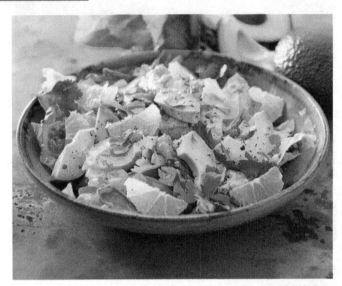

Crispy Romaine and Avocado Citrus Salad

Prep: 10 minutes | Cook: 0 minutes | Serves: 2

Ingredients:

- 4 cups chopped romaine lettuce (200g)
- 1 medium avocado, diced (150g)
- 1/2 cup orange segments (120g)
- 2 tbsp extra-virgin olive oil (30ml)
- 1 tbsp fresh lime juice (15ml)
- 1 tsp Dijon mustard (5g)
- 1/4 tsp salt (1g)
- 1/4 tsp black pepper (1g)
- 2 tbsp chopped fresh cilantro (8g)

Instructions:

1. Place the romaine lettuce in a large salad bowl and top with diced avocado and orange segments.
2. In a small bowl, whisk together olive oil, lime juice, Dijon mustard, salt, and black pepper to make the dressing.
3. Drizzle the dressing over the salad and toss gently to combine.
4. Sprinkle the chopped cilantro over the salad as garnish.

Nutritional Facts (Per Serving): Calories: 380 | Fat: 15g | Carbs: 42g | Fiber: 9g | Sugars: 9g | Protein: 10g | Sodium: 320mg

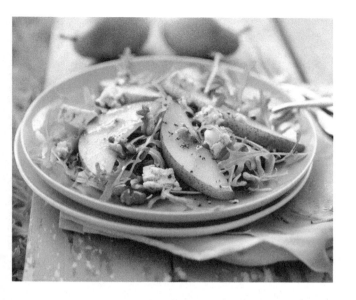

Arugula, Pear & Gorgonzola Crunch

Prep: 10 minutes | Cook: 0 minutes | Serves: 2

Ingredients:

- 4 cups arugula (120g)
- 1 medium pear, thinly sliced (150g)
- 1/4 cup crumbled Gorgonzola cheese (30g)
- 1/4 cup chopped walnuts, toasted (30g)
- 2 tbsp olive oil (30ml)
- 1 tbsp balsamic vinegar (15ml)
- 1 tsp Dijon mustard (5g)
- 1/4 tsp salt (1g)
- 1/4 tsp black pepper (1g)

Instructions:

1. Place arugula in a large salad bowl and top with sliced pear, crumbled Gorgonzola, and toasted walnuts.
2. In a small bowl, whisk together olive oil, balsamic vinegar, Dijon mustard, salt, and black pepper to make the dressing.
3. Drizzle the dressing over the salad and toss gently to combine.
4. Divide the salad between two plates for serving.
5. Enjoy immediately for a fresh, crunchy bite.

Nutritional Facts (Per Serving): Calories: 380 | Fat: 17g | Carbs: 42g | Fiber: 7g | Sugars: 12g | Protein: 9g | Sodium: 350mg

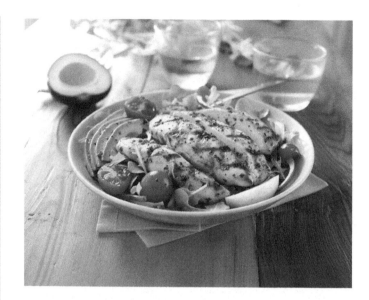

Zesty Lemon Herb Grilled Chicken Salad

Prep: 15 minutes | Cook: 15 minutes | Serves: 2

Ingredients:

- 2 chicken breasts, boneless and skinless (5 oz each) (140g each)
- 4 cups mixed greens (120g)
- 1/2 cup cherry tomatoes, halved (75g)
- 1/4 cup sliced red onion (30g)
- 1/2 avocado, sliced (75g)
- 2 tbsp olive oil (30ml)
- 2 tbsp fresh lemon juice (30ml)
- 1 tsp fresh lemon zest (2g)
- 1 tsp dried oregano (2g)
- 1/4 tsp salt (1g)
- 1/4 tsp black pepper (1g)

Instructions:

1. Preheat a grill to medium heat.
2. Rub chicken breasts with 1 tbsp olive oil, lemon zest, oregano, salt, and pepper. Grill for 6-7 minutes per side until fully cooked.
3. While the chicken rests, arrange mixed greens, cherry tomatoes, red onion, and avocado slices in a salad bowl.
4. In a small bowl, whisk together the remaining olive oil and lemon juice to make the dressing.
5. Slice the grilled chicken, place it on the salad, drizzle with dressing, and serve.

Nutritional Facts (Per Serving): Calories: 380 | Fat: 15g | Carbs: 12g | Fiber: 5g | Sugars: 4g | Protein: 38g | Sodium: 360mg

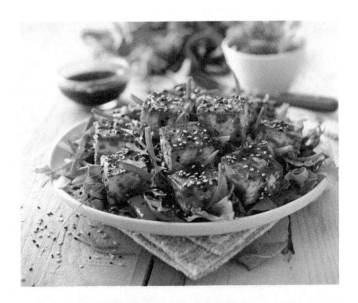

Asian Sesame Tofu & Veggie Salad

Prep: 15 minutes | Cook: 10 minutes | Serves: 2

Ingredients:

- 1 block firm tofu, cubed (8 oz) (225g)
- 4 cups mixed greens (120g)
- 1 cup shredded carrots (100g)
- 1 cup sliced red bell peppers (100g)
- 2 tbsp sesame oil (30ml)
- 1 tbsp low-sodium soy sauce (15ml)
- 1 tsp grated fresh ginger (5g)
- 1 tsp sesame seeds (5g)
- 1 tbsp rice vinegar (15ml)
- 1/4 tsp black pepper (1g)

Instructions:

1. Heat 1 tbsp sesame oil in a skillet over medium heat. Add tofu cubes and cook until golden brown, 3-4 minutes per side.
2. In a small bowl, whisk together the remaining sesame oil, soy sauce, ginger, rice vinegar, and black pepper to make the dressing.
3. Arrange mixed greens, carrots, and red bell peppers on a plate.
4. Top with the cooked tofu and drizzle with the sesame dressing.
5. Sprinkle sesame seeds on top and serve immediately.

Nutritional Facts (Per Serving): Calories: 380 | Fat: 18g | Carbs: 20g | Fiber: 5g | Sugars: 6g | Protein: 19g | Sodium: 350mg

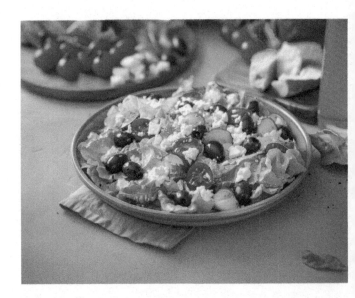

Greek Goddess Salad with Feta & Olives

Prep: 10 minutes | Cook: 0 minutes | Serves: 2

Ingredients:

- 4 cups chopped romaine lettuce (200g)
- 1/2 cup cherry tomatoes, halved (75g)
- 1/4 cup sliced cucumber (50g)
- 1/4 cup crumbled feta cheese (30g)
- 1/4 cup Kalamata olives, pitted and halved (30g)
- 2 tbsp olive oil (30ml)
- 1 tbsp fresh lemon juice (15ml)
- 1 tsp dried oregano (2g)
- 1/4 tsp salt (1g)
- 1/4 tsp black pepper (1g)

Instructions:

1. Place romaine lettuce in a large salad bowl and layer with cherry tomatoes, cucumber slices, feta cheese, and Kalamata olives.
2. In a small bowl, whisk together olive oil, lemon juice, oregano, salt, and black pepper to make the dressing.
3. Drizzle the dressing over the salad and toss gently to combine.
4. Divide the salad between two plates for serving.
5. Enjoy fresh with crusty whole-grain bread, if desired.

Nutritional Facts (Per Serving): Calories: 380 | Fat: 16g | Carbs: 22g | Fiber: 6g | Sugars: 5g | Protein: 13g | Sodium: 370mg

CHAPTER 16: DINNER: Fiber-Rich Vegetable Mains For A Satisfying Meal

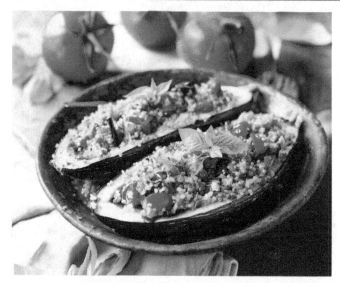

Eggplant and Quinoa Stuffed Zucchini Boats

Prep: 15 minutes | Cook: 25 minutes | Serves: 2

Ingredients:

- 2 medium zucchinis, halved lengthwise (8 oz each) (225g each)
- 1/2 cup cooked quinoa (85g)
- 1/2 cup diced eggplant (75g)
- 1/4 cup diced tomatoes (60g)
- 2 tbsp olive oil (30ml)
- 1 tbsp grated Parmesan cheese (15g)
- 1 tsp dried oregano (2g)
- 1/2 tsp garlic powder (1g)
- 1/4 tsp salt (1g)
- 1/4 tsp black pepper (1g)

Instructions:

1. Preheat oven to 375°F (190°C). Scoop out the centers of the zucchini halves to create boats and set aside.
2. Heat 1 tbsp olive oil in a skillet over medium heat. Sauté diced eggplant and tomatoes with oregano, garlic powder, salt, and pepper for 5 minutes.
3. Stir in cooked quinoa and cook for 2 minutes.
4. Fill the zucchini with the mixture, drizzle with remaining olive oil, sprinkle with Parmesan, and bake for 20 minutes until tender. Serve warm.

Nutritional Facts (Per Serving): Calories: 380 | Fat: 16g | Carbs: 42g | Fiber: 8g | Sugars: 6g | Protein: 12g | Sodium: 380mg

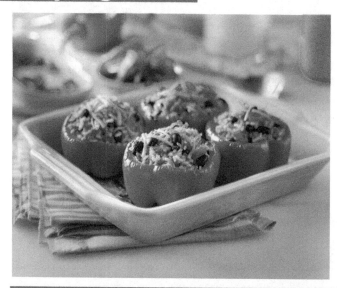

Stuffed Bell Peppers with Black Beans and Brown Rice

Prep: 15 minutes | Cook: 25 minutes | Serves: 2

Ingredients:

- 2 large bell peppers, halved and cored (6 oz each) (170g each)
- 1/2 cup cooked brown rice (85g)
- 1/2 cup cooked black beans (85g)
- 1/4 cup diced tomatoes (60g)
- 2 tbsp shredded cheddar cheese (30g)
- 1 tbsp olive oil (15ml)
- 1 tsp chili powder (2g)
- 1/2 tsp cumin (1g)
- 1/4 tsp salt (1g)
- 1/4 tsp black pepper (1g)

Instructions:

1. Preheat oven to 375°F (190°C). Place bell pepper halves in a baking dish.
2. In a bowl, mix cooked brown rice, black beans, diced tomatoes, chili powder, cumin, salt, pepper.
3. Stuff the bell pepper halves with the rice mixture and drizzle with olive oil.
4. Sprinkle shredded cheddar cheese on top of each pepper.
5. Bake for 25 minutes until the peppers are tender and the cheese is melted. Serve warm.

Nutritional Facts (Per Serving): Calories: 380 | Fat: 12g | Carbs: 48g | Fiber: 9g | Sugars: 6g | Protein: 13g | Sodium: 370mg

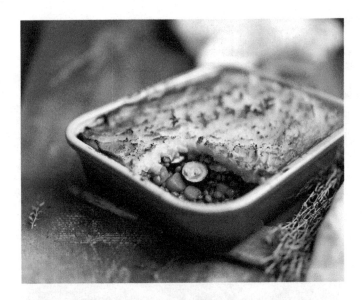

Roasted Vegetable and Lentil Shepherd's Pie

Prep: 20 minutes | Cook: 30 minutes | Serves: 2

Ingredients:

- 1 cup cooked lentils (170g)
- 1 cup diced carrots (120g)
- 1 cup diced zucchini (120g)
- 1 cup diced mushrooms (100g)
- 2 tbsp olive oil (30ml)
- 1 tbsp tomato paste (15g)
- 1/2 tsp dried thyme (1g)
- 1/4 tsp salt (1g)
- 1/4 tsp black pepper (1g)
- 2 cups mashed potatoes (300g), made with low-fat milk

Instructions:

1. Preheat oven to 375°F (190°C). Roast diced carrots, zucchini, and mushrooms with 1 tbsp olive oil for 15 minutes.
2. Heat the remaining olive oil in a skillet. Add lentils, tomato paste, thyme, salt, and pepper. Cook for 5 minutes.
3. Stir the roasted vegetables into the lentil mixture.
4. Spread the mixture in a baking dish and top with mashed potatoes. Smooth with a spatula.
5. Bake for 20 minutes until golden. Let cool slightly before serving.

Nutritional Facts (Per Serving): Calories: 380 | Fat: 10g | Carbs: 55g | Fiber: 9g | Sugars: 7g | Protein: 12g | Sodium: 380mg

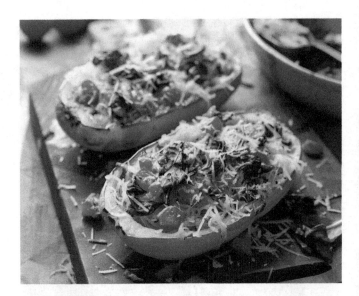

Spaghetti Squash with Tomato Basil and Spinach

Prep: 15 minutes | Cook: 25 minutes | Serves: 2

Ingredients:

- 1 medium spaghetti squash, halved (4 cups cooked) (600g)
- 1 cup diced tomatoes (150g)
- 1 cup fresh spinach, chopped (30g)
- 2 tbsp olive oil (30ml)
- 2 tbsp fresh basil, chopped (8g)
- 1 clove garlic, minced (3g)
- 1/4 tsp salt (1g)
- 1/4 tsp black pepper (1g)
- 2 tbsp grated Parmesan cheese (15g)

Instructions:

1. Preheat oven to 400°F (200°C). Roast spaghetti squash halves face down for 20 minutes. Scrape out the strands with a fork.
2. Heat olive oil in a skillet. Sauté garlic for 1 minute, then add diced tomatoes and spinach. Cook for 5 minutes.
3. Stir in the spaghetti squash strands and toss to combine. Season with salt and pepper.
4. Remove from heat and mix in fresh basil.
5. Serve topped with grated Parmesan cheese.

Nutritional Facts (Per Serving): Calories: 380 | Fat: 12g | Carbs: 46g | Fiber: 8g | Sugars: 8g | Protein: 10g | Sodium: 350mg

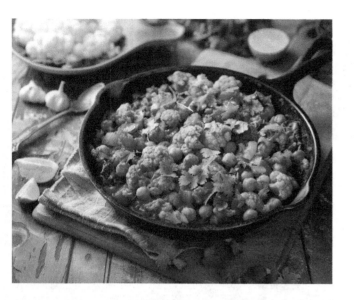

Cauliflower and Chickpea Tikka Masala

Prep: 15 minutes | Cook: 25 minutes | Serves: 2

Ingredients:

- 2 cups cauliflower florets (200g)
- 1 cup cooked chickpeas (170g)
- 1 cup diced tomatoes (150g)
- 1/2 cup unsweetened coconut milk (120ml)
- 1/2 cup diced onion (75g)
- 2 tbsp olive oil (30ml)
- 1 tbsp tikka masala spice blend (6g)
- 1 clove garlic, minced (3g)
- 1/4 tsp salt (1g)
- 2 tbsp chopped fresh cilantro (8g)

Instructions:

1. Heat olive oil in a large skillet over medium heat. Sauté diced onion and garlic for 2 minutes.
2. Add tikka masala spice blend and cook for 1 minute until fragrant.
3. Stir in cauliflower, chickpeas, diced tomatoes, and coconut milk. Season with salt.
4. Cover and simmer for 15 minutes, stirring occasionally, until the cauliflower is tender.
5. Garnish with chopped cilantro.
6. Serve warm.

Nutritional Facts (Per Serving): Calories: 380 | Fat: 14g | Carbs: 47g | Fiber: 9g | Sugars: 6g | Protein: 12g | Sodium: 360mg

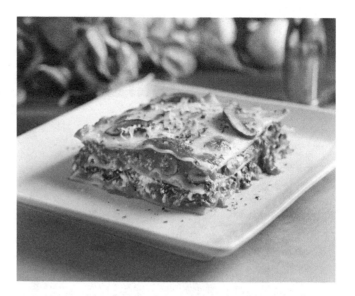

Mushroom and Spinach Whole Wheat Lasagna

Prep: 20 minutes | Cook: 30 minutes | Serves: 2

Ingredients:

- 4 whole wheat lasagna sheets (100g)
- 1 cup sliced mushrooms (100g)
- 1 cup fresh spinach, chopped (30g)
- 1 cup low-fat ricotta cheese (240g)
- 1/2 cup shredded mozzarella cheese (60g)
- 1/2 cup low-sodium marinara sauce (120ml)
- 1 tbsp olive oil (15ml)
- 1/4 tsp dried oregano (1g)
- 1/4 tsp salt (1g)
- 1/4 tsp black pepper (1g)

Instructions:

1. Preheat oven to 375°F (190°C). Cook lasagna sheets according to package instructions.
2. Heat olive oil in a skillet. Sauté mushrooms with oregano, salt, and pepper for 5 minutes. Stir in spinach and cook until wilted.
3. In a baking dish, spread a thin layer of marinara sauce. Layer lasagna sheets, mushroom-spinach mixture, ricotta, and marinara sauce, repeating until ingredients are used.
4. Top with shredded mozzarella cheese.
5. Bake for 20 minutes until bubbly and golden. Serve warm.

Nutritional Facts (Per Serving): Calories: 380 | Fat: 13g | Carbs: 43g | Fiber: 8g | Sugars: 5g | Protein: 17g | Sodium: 380mg

CHAPTER 17: DINNER: Heart-Smart Fish And Seafood Dishes With Dash-Approved Herbs And Spices

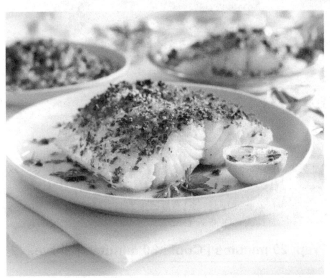

Herb-Crusted Baked Cod with Lemon Zest

Prep: 10 minutes | Cook: 20 minutes | Serves: 2

Ingredients:

- 2 cod fillets (5 oz each) (140g each)
- 1/4 cup whole wheat breadcrumbs (30g)
- 2 tbsp chopped fresh parsley (8g)
- 1 tbsp olive oil (15ml)
- 1 tsp lemon zest (2g)
- 1/2 tsp dried thyme (1g)
- 1/4 tsp salt (1g)
- 1/4 tsp black pepper (1g)

Instructions:

1. Preheat oven to 375°F (190°C). Line a baking sheet with parchment paper.
2. In a bowl, mix breadcrumbs, parsley, olive oil, lemon zest, thyme, salt, and pepper to create the herb crust.
3. Place cod fillets on the prepared baking sheet and press the herb mixture onto the top of each fillet. Bake for 18-20 minutes until the cod is flaky and golden on top.
4. Serve with a wedge of lemon for extra zest.

Nutritional Facts (Per Serving): Calories: 380 | Fat: 12g | Carbs: 18g | Fiber: 2g | Sugars: 1g | Protein: 45g | Sodium: 380mg

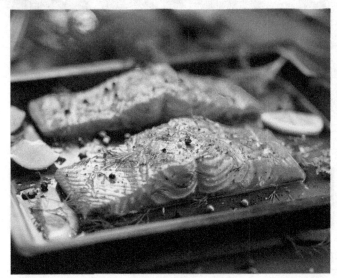

Garlic and Dill Salmon Fillets

Prep: 10 minutes | Cook: 15 minutes | Serves: 2

Ingredients:

- 2 salmon fillets (6 oz each) (170g each)
- 1 tbsp olive oil (15ml)
- 2 cloves garlic, minced (6g)
- 1 tbsp fresh dill, chopped (4g)
- Juice of 1/2 lemon (15ml)
- 1/4 tsp salt (1g)
- 1/4 tsp black pepper (1g)

Instructions:

1. Preheat oven to 400°F (200°C). Line a baking dish with foil.
2. In a small bowl, mix olive oil, minced garlic, dill, lemon juice, salt, and pepper.
3. Place salmon fillets in the baking dish and brush the garlic-dill mixture evenly over each fillet.
4. Bake for 12-15 minutes until the salmon is cooked through and flakes easily with a fork.
5. Serve immediately with a side of steamed vegetables or a green salad.

Nutritional Facts (Per Serving): Calories: 380 | Fat: 18g | Carbs: 2g | Fiber: 0g | Sugars: 0g | Protein: 45g | Sodium: 360mg

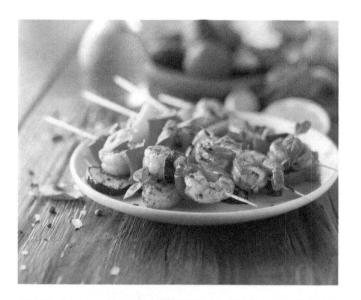

Spiced Shrimp and Vegetable Skewers

Prep: 15 minutes | Cook: 10 minutes | Serves: 2

Ingredients:

- 8 oz large shrimp, peeled and deveined (225g)
- 1 cup zucchini slices (120g)
- 1 cup bell pepper chunks (120g)
- 1 cup cherry tomatoes (150g)
- 2 tbsp olive oil (30ml)
- 1 tsp smoked paprika (2g)
- 1/2 tsp garlic powder (1g)
- 1/4 tsp cayenne pepper (1g)
- 1/4 tsp salt (1g)
- 1/4 tsp black pepper (1g)

Instructions:

1. Preheat grill or grill pan to medium heat.
2. In a bowl, toss shrimp and vegetables with olive oil, smoked paprika, garlic powder, cayenne pepper, salt, and black pepper.
3. Thread shrimp and vegetables onto skewers, alternating for even distribution.
4. Grill skewers for 3-4 minutes per side until shrimp are pink and cooked through.
5. Serve immediately with a side of mixed greens or quinoa.

Nutritional Facts (Per Serving): Calories: 380 | Fat: 14g | Carbs: 16g | Fiber: 4g | Sugars: 7g | Protein: 36g | Sodium: 380mg

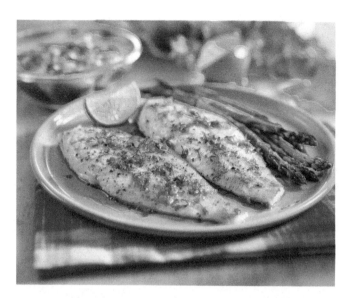

Cilantro Lime Tilapia with Steamed Asparagus

Prep: 10 minutes | Cook: 15 minutes | Serves: 2

Ingredients:

- 2 tilapia fillets (5 oz each) (140g each)
- 1/2 cup fresh cilantro, chopped (15g)
- Juice and zest of 1 lime (15ml juice, 2g zest)
- 2 tbsp olive oil (30ml)
- 1 clove garlic, minced (3g)
- 1/4 tsp salt (1g)
- 1/4 tsp black pepper (1g)
- 1 cup asparagus spears, trimmed (150g)

Instructions:

1. Preheat oven to 375°F (190°C). Place tilapia fillets on a lined baking sheet.
2. In a small bowl, mix cilantro, lime juice, lime zest, olive oil, garlic, salt, and pepper. Brush the mixture over the tilapia.
3. Bake for 12-15 minutes until the fish flakes easily with a fork.
4. Steam asparagus in a steamer basket over boiling water for 5-7 minutes until tender.
5. Serve tilapia with steamed asparagus on the side.

Nutritional Facts (Per Serving): Calories: 380 | Fat: 13g | Carbs: 10g | Fiber: 3g | Sugars: 2g | Protein: 48g | Sodium: 350mg

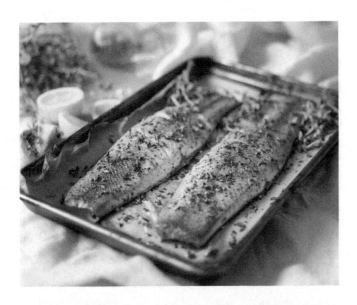

Paprika and Thyme Baked Trout

Prep: 10 minutes | Cook: 15 minutes | Serves: 2

Ingredients:

- 2 trout fillets (6 oz each) (170g each)
- 1 tbsp olive oil (15ml)
- 1 tsp smoked paprika (2g)
- 1 tsp fresh thyme leaves (1g)
- 1/2 tsp garlic powder (1g)
- 1/4 tsp salt (1g)
- 1/4 tsp black pepper (1g)
- Juice of 1/2 lemon (15ml)

Instructions:

1. Preheat oven to 375°F (190°C). Line a baking sheet with parchment paper.
2. Rub trout fillets with olive oil, smoked paprika, thyme, garlic powder, salt, and black pepper.
3. Place the trout fillets on the prepared baking sheet and drizzle with lemon juice.
4. Bake for 12-15 minutes until the trout is flaky and cooked through.
5. Serve immediately with a side of steamed greens or a fresh salad.

Nutritional Facts (Per Serving): Calories: 380 | Fat: 15g | Carbs: 2g | Fiber: 0g | Sugars: 0g | Protein: 50g | Sodium: 360mg

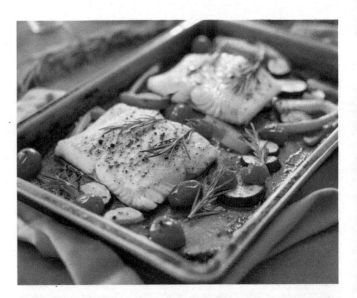

Rosemary Lemon Baked Haddock with Roasted Vegetables

Prep: 15 minutes | Cook: 20 minutes | Serves: 2

Ingredients:

- 2 haddock fillets (6 oz each) (170g each)
- 1 cup zucchini slices (120g)
- 1 cup bell pepper chunks (120g)
- 1 cup cherry tomatoes (150g)
- 2 tbsp olive oil (30ml)
- 1 tbsp fresh rosemary, chopped (4g)
- Juice and zest of 1 lemon (15ml juice, 2g zest)
- 1/4 tsp salt (1g)
- 1/4 tsp black pepper (1g)

Instructions:

1. Preheat oven to 400°F (200°C). Line a baking sheet with parchment paper.
2. Toss zucchini, bell peppers, and cherry tomatoes with 1 tbsp olive oil, salt, and black pepper. Spread on one side of the baking sheet.
3. Place haddock fillets on the other side. Drizzle with remaining olive oil, lemon juice, and zest, then sprinkle with rosemary.
4. Bake for 18-20 minutes until the haddock is flaky and vegetables are tender.
5. Serve the haddock alongside the roasted vegetables.

Nutritional Facts (Per Serving): Calories: 380 | Fat: 14g | Carbs: 12g | Fiber: 4g | Sugars: 5g | Protein: 45g | Sodium: 370mg

CHAPTER 18: DINNER: Special Occasion Meals That Celebrate Without Compromising Heart Health

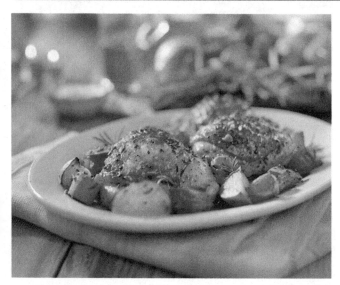

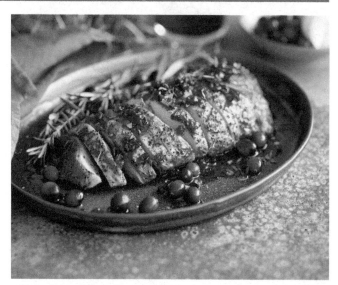

Rosemary and Garlic Roast Chicken with Root Vegetables

Prep: 15 minutes | Cook: 40 minutes | Serves: 2

Ingredients:

- 2 chicken thighs, skinless (6 oz each) (170g each)
- 1 cup diced carrots (120g)
- 1 cup diced parsnips (120g)
- 1 cup diced sweet potatoes (150g)
- 2 tbsp olive oil (30ml)
- 1 tsp fresh rosemary, chopped (2g)
- 2 cloves garlic, minced (6g)
- 1/4 tsp salt (1g)
- 1/4 tsp black pepper (1g)

Instructions:

1. Preheat oven to 375°F (190°C). Place chicken thighs in a baking dish.
2. In a bowl, toss carrots, parsnips, and potatoes with olive oil, rosemary, garlic, salt, and pepper.
3. Arrange the seasoned vegetables around the chicken in the dish. Drizzle remaining olive oil over the chicken.
4. Roast for 35-40 minutes until the chicken is fully cooked (165°F/74°C internal temperature) and vegetables are tender.
5. Serve chicken with the roasted vegetables.

Nutritional Facts (Per Serving): Calories: 380 | Fat: 15g | Carbs: 30g | Fiber: 6g | Sugars: 8g | Protein: 35g | Sodium: 380mg

Herb-Infused Turkey Breast with Cranberry Glaze

Prep: 15 minutes | Cook: 30 minutes | Serves: 2

Ingredients:

- 2 turkey breast (5 oz each) (140g each)
- 1/2 cup fresh cranberries (50g)
- 1 tbsp honey (20g)
- 1/4 cup chicken broth, low-sodium (60ml)
- 1 tbsp olive oil (15ml)
- 1 tsp dried thyme (2g)
- 1/2 tsp garlic powder (1g)
- 1/4 tsp salt (1g)
- 1/4 tsp black pepper (1g)

Instructions:

1. Preheat oven to 375°F (190°C). Rub turkey with olive oil, thyme, garlic powder, salt, and black pepper.
2. Heat a skillet over medium heat and sear turkey for 2 minutes per side. Transfer to a baking dish.
3. In a saucepan, combine cranberries, honey, and chicken broth. Simmer for 5 minutes until cranberries burst, forming a glaze.
4. Pour the cranberry glaze over the turkey and bake for 20-25 minutes.
5. Serve the turkey with a drizzle of the glaze and a side of steamed green beans or a salad.

Nutritional Facts (Per Serving): Calories: 380 | Fat: 10g | Carbs: 18g | Fiber: 2g | Sugars: 8g | Protein: 50g | Sodium: 360mg

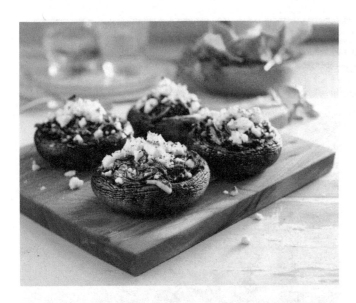

Stuffed Portobello Mushrooms with Spinach and Feta

Prep: 15 minutes | Cook: 20 minutes | Serves: 2

Ingredients:

- 4 large Portobello mushrooms, stems removed (7 oz each) (200g each)
- 2 cups fresh spinach, chopped (60g)
- 1/4 cup crumbled feta cheese (30g)
- 2 tbsp olive oil (30ml)
- 1 clove garlic, minced (3g)
- 1 tsp dried oregano (2g)
- 1/4 tsp salt (1g)
- 1/4 tsp black pepper (1g)

Instructions:

1. Preheat oven to 375°F (190°C). Brush Portobello caps with olive oil and place them on a baking sheet.
2. In a skillet, heat 1 tbsp olive oil over medium heat. Sauté garlic and spinach for 2-3 minutes until wilted. Season with oregano, salt, and pepper.
3. Fill each mushroom cap with the spinach mixture and top with crumbled feta cheese.
4. Bake for 15-20 minutes until the mushrooms are tender and the feta is slightly golden.
5. Serve warm with a side salad or steamed vegetables.

Nutritional Facts (Per Serving): Calories: 380 | Fat: 15g | Carbs: 25g | Fiber: 7g | Sugars: 6g | Protein: 22g | Sodium: 380mg

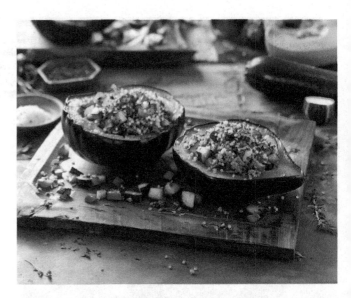

Vegetable-Stuffed Acorn Squash with Quinoa Pilaf

Prep: 15 minutes | Cook: 30 minutes | Serves: 2

Ingredients:

- 1 medium acorn squash, halved and seeded (22 oz) (620g)
- 1/2 cup cooked quinoa (85g)
- 1/2 cup diced zucchini (60g)
- 1/2 cup diced red bell pepper (60g)
- 1/4 cup diced onion (40g)
- 2 tbsp olive oil (30ml)
- 1 tsp dried thyme (2g)
- 1/4 tsp salt (1g)
- 1/4 tsp black pepper (1g)

Instructions:

1. Preheat oven to 375°F (190°C). Brush acorn squash halves with 1 tbsp olive oil and roast cut-side down for 20 minutes.
2. In a skillet, heat 1 tbsp olive oil. Sauté onion, zucchini, and bell pepper for 5 minutes. Stir in quinoa, thyme, salt, and pepper.
3. Fill roasted squash halves with the quinoa-vegetable mixture.
4. Return to the oven and bake for 10 minutes.
5. Serve warm, garnished with fresh herbs if desired.

Nutritional Facts (Per Serving): Calories: 380 | Fat: 13g | Carbs: 53g | Fiber: 9g | Sugars: 8g | Protein: 10g | Sodium: 350mg

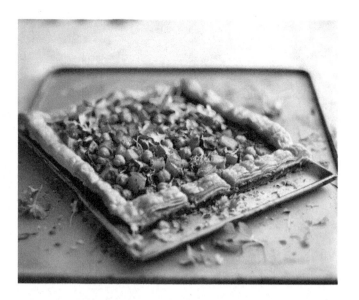

Moroccan Spiced Vegetable and Chickpea Tart

Prep: 20 minutes | Cook: 25 minutes | Serves: 2

Ingredients:

- 1 sheet whole wheat puff pastry (6 oz) (170g)
- 1 cup cooked chickpeas (170g)
- 1/2 cup diced eggplant (75g)
- 1/2 cup diced zucchini (75g)
- 1/4 cup diced red bell pepper (40g)
- 2 tbsp olive oil (30ml)
- 1 tsp ground cumin (2g)
- 1 tsp ground coriander (2g)
- 1/2 tsp smoked paprika (1g)
- 1/4 tsp salt (1g)
- 1/4 tsp black pepper (1g)

Instructions:

1. Preheat oven to 375°F (190°C). Roll out puff pastry on a baking sheet and fold edges to create a border.
2. Heat olive oil in a skillet and sauté eggplant, zucchini, and bell pepper for 5 minutes. Add chickpeas and spices, stirring for 2 minutes.
3. Spread the vegetable mixture evenly over the puff pastry.
4. Bake for 20-25 minutes until the pastry is golden brown.
5. Serve warm, garnished with fresh parsley or cilantro.

Nutritional Facts (Per Serving): Calories: 380 | Fat: 14g | Carbs: 48g | Fiber: 8g | Sugars: 6g | Protein: 10g | Sodium: 350mg

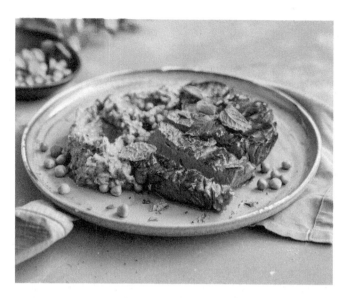

Garlic and Herb Roasted Lamb with Minted Pea Puree

Prep: 15 minutes | Cook: 25 minutes | Serves: 2

Ingredients:

- 2 lamb loin chops (5 oz each) (140g each)
- 1 tbsp olive oil (15ml)
- 2 cloves garlic, minced (6g)
- 1 tsp fresh rosemary, chopped (2g)
- 1/4 tsp salt (1g)
- 1/4 tsp black pepper (1g)
- 1 cup fresh peas (150g)
- 1 tbsp fresh mint, chopped (4g)
- 1/4 cup low-fat milk (60ml)

Instructions:

1. Preheat oven to 400°F (200°C). Rub lamb chops with olive oil, garlic, rosemary, salt, and pepper.
2. Sear lamb chops in a hot skillet for 2 minutes per side, then transfer to the oven to roast for 15 minutes.
3. Boil peas for 5 minutes, then drain and puree with mint and milk until smooth. Season with salt and pepper.
4. Let lamb rest for 5 minutes before serving.
5. Serve lamb chops with minted pea puree on the side.

Nutritional Facts (Per Serving): Calories: 380 | Fat: 15g | Carbs: 12g | Fiber: 4g | Sugars: 4g | Protein: 45g | Sodium: 360mg

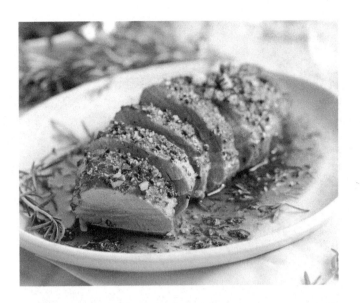

Herb-Crusted Pork Tenderloin with Apple Cider Reduction

Prep: 15 minutes | Cook: 25 minutes | Serves: 2

Ingredients:

- 1 pork tenderloin (12 oz) (340g)
- 2 tbsp olive oil (30ml)
- 1 tbsp fresh rosemary, chopped (4g)
- 1 tsp dried thyme (2g)
- 1 clove garlic, minced (3g)
- 1/4 tsp salt (1g)
- 1/4 tsp black pepper (1g)
- 1/2 cup apple cider (120ml)
- 1 tsp Dijon mustard (5g)

Instructions:

1. Preheat oven to 400°F (200°C). Rub pork tenderloin with 1 tbsp olive oil, rosemary, thyme, garlic, salt, and black pepper.
2. Heat 1 tbsp olive oil in an oven-safe skillet and sear pork for 2 minutes per side.
3. Transfer skillet to the oven and roast for 18-20 minutes until the internal temperature reaches 145°F (63°C).
4. In the same skillet, simmer apple cider and Dijon mustard for 5 minutes until reduced by half.
5. Slice pork, drizzle with the apple cider reduction, and serve.

Nutritional Facts (Per Serving): Calories: 380 | Fat: 14g | Carbs: 12g | Fiber: 0g | Sugars: 8g | Protein: 45g | Sodium: 360mg

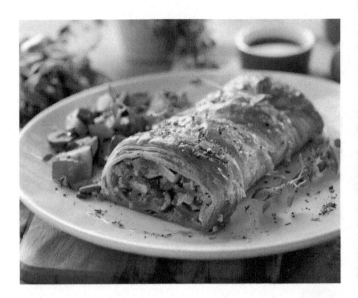

Vegetable Wellington with Whole Grain Puff Pastry

Prep: 20 minutes | Cook: 30 minutes | Serves: 2

Ingredients:

- 1 sheet whole grain puff pastry (6 oz) (170g)
- 1 cup diced mushrooms (100g)
- 1/2 cup diced zucchini (60g)
- 1/2 cup diced red bell pepper (60g)
- 1/4 cup diced onion (40g)
- 2 tbsp olive oil (30ml)
- 1 tsp dried thyme (2g)
- 1/4 tsp salt (1g)
- 1/4 tsp black pepper (1g)
- 1 egg, beaten (50g)

Instructions:

1. Preheat oven to 375°F (190°C). Heat olive oil in a skillet and sauté onion, mushrooms, zucchini, and bell pepper for 5 minutes. Stir in thyme, salt, and pepper. Let cool.
2. Roll out puff pastry on a baking sheet and spread the vegetable mixture in the center.
3. Fold the pastry over the filling, sealing the edges. Brush with beaten egg.
4. Bake for 25-30 minutes until golden brown.
5. Slice and serve warm with a side salad.

Nutritional Facts (Per Serving): Calories: 380 | Fat: 15g | Carbs: 45g | Fiber: 7g | Sugars: 5g | Protein: 10g | Sodium: 350mg

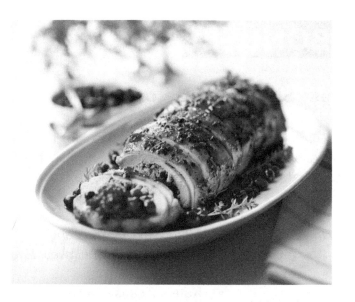

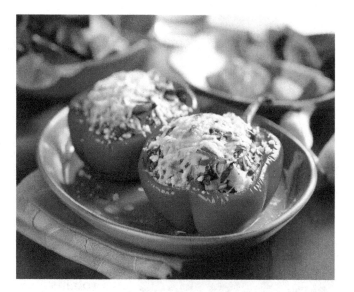

Maple Dijon Glazed Turkey Roulade with Cranberry Relish

Prep: 20 minutes | Cook: 30 minutes | Serves: 2

Ingredients:

- 2 turkey breast cutlets (5 oz each) (140g each)
- 2 tbsp Dijon mustard (30g)
- 1 tbsp maple syrup (20ml)
- 1 tsp dried thyme (2g)
- 1/4 tsp salt (1g)
- 1/4 tsp black pepper (1g)
- 1/2 cup fresh cranberries (50g)
- 1 tbsp honey (15g)
- 1/4 cup water (60ml)

Instructions:

1. Preheat oven to 375°F (190°C). Pound turkey cutlets to an even thickness.
2. Mix Dijon mustard, maple syrup, thyme, salt, and pepper. Spread over each cutlet, roll tightly, and secure with toothpicks.
3. Bake for 25-30 minutes until the internal temperature reaches 165°F (74°C).
4. In a saucepan, simmer cranberries, honey, and water for 5 minutes until thickened into a relish.
5. Slice turkey roulade, drizzle with cranberry relish, and serve.

Nutritional Facts (Per Serving): Calories: 380 | Fat: 10g | Carbs: 18g | Fiber: 2g | Sugars: 10g | Protein: 50g | Sodium: 360mg

Spinach and Artichoke Stuffed Bell Peppers

Prep: 15 minutes | Cook: 25 minutes | Serves: 2

Ingredients:

- 2 large bell peppers, halved and cored (6 oz each) (170g each)
- 1 cup fresh spinach, chopped (30g)
- 1/2 cup diced artichoke hearts (75g)
- 1/4 cup low-fat ricotta cheese (60g)
- 2 tbsp grated Parmesan cheese (15g)
- 1 tbsp olive oil (15ml)
- 1 clove garlic, minced (3g)
- 1/4 tsp salt (1g)
- 1/4 tsp black pepper (1g)

Instructions:

1. Preheat oven to 375°F (190°C). Place bell pepper halves in a baking dish.
2. Heat olive oil in a skillet and sauté garlic, spinach, and artichoke hearts for 3-4 minutes. Remove from heat and stir in ricotta, Parmesan, salt, and pepper.
3. Stuff each pepper half with the spinach-artichoke mixture.
4. Bake for 20-25 minutes until peppers are tender.
5. Serve warm with a side of mixed greens or quinoa.

Nutritional Facts (Per Serving): Calories: 380 | Fat: 13g | Carbs: 25g | Fiber: 6g | Sugars: 6g | Protein: 25g | Sodium: 350mg

CHAPTER 19: BONUSES

Meal Plans and Shopping Templates: Simplified Keto Planning

This cookbook includes a 30-day grocery shopping guide tailored for one person. It's designed to simplify your keto journey by focusing on fresh, high-quality ingredients and minimizing processed foods. Be mindful of hidden carbs in condiments and dressings, and adjust quantities to suit your dietary needs. Enjoy a seamless transition to flavorful, keto-friendly cooking!

Grocery Shopping List for 7-Day Meal Plan

Grains & Legumes

- **Quinoa** – 2 cups / 360 g (*Quinoa Tropical Mango Coconut Porridge, Grilled Chicken and Quinoa Salad, Vegetable-Stuffed Acorn Squash with Quinoa Pilaf*)
- **Steel-Cut Oats** – 1 cup / 180 g (*Steel-Cut Oat Maple Pecan Pumpkin Porridge*)
- **Whole Wheat Flour** – 1 cup / 120 g (*Whole Wheat Blueberry Pancakes*)
- **Brown Rice** – 1 cup / 180 g (*Mushroom and Pea Brown Rice Risotto*)
- **Farro** – 1 cup / 180 g (*Herbed Chicken and Farro Pilaf*)
- **Lentils** – 1 cup / 200 g (*Lentil and Vegetable Stuffed Eggplant*)
- **White Beans (canned)** – 1 can / 400 g (*Tuscan White Bean Minestrone*)
- **Chickpeas (canned)** – 1 can / 400 g (*Moroccan Chickpea and Spinach Soup, Vegetable-Stuffed*

Acorn Squash with Quinoa Pilaf)

Proteins

- **Eggs** – 14 large (*Avocado and Egg Breakfast Bowl, Southwest Egg Muffins, Mediterranean Veggie Omelette*)
- **Greek Yogurt (plain, unsweetened)** – 3 cups / 720 g (*Greek Yogurt Parfait with Fresh Fruits*)
- **Chicken Breast** – 2 fillets / 12 oz / 340 g (*Grilled Chicken and Quinoa Salad, Herbed Chicken and Farro Pilaf*)
- **Salmon Fillets** – 2 fillets / 10 oz / 280 g (*Garlic and Dill Salmon Fillets*)
- **Cod Fillets** – 1 fillet / 8 oz / 225 g (*Herb-Crusted Baked Cod with Lemon Zest*)
- **Lamb (boneless)** – 1 lb / 450 g (*Garlic and Herb Roasted Lamb with Minted Pea Puree*)
- **Shrimp** – 8 oz / 225 g (*Spiced Shrimp and Vegetable Skewers*)

Vegetables

- **Spinach (fresh)** – 6 cups / 180 g (*Spinach and Artichoke Stuffed Bell Peppers,*

Moroccan Chickpea and Spinach Soup, Southwest Egg Muffins)
- **Kale** – 2 cups / 100 g (*Citrus Kale and Orange Smoothie*)
- **Mushrooms** – 3 cups / 300 g (*Mushroom and Spinach Whole Wheat Lasagna, Mushroom and Pea Brown Rice Risotto*)
- **Bell Peppers** – 4 large (*Spinach and Artichoke Stuffed Bell Peppers, Southwest Egg Muffins*)
- **Zucchini** – 2 medium (*Zesty Lemon Herb Tzatziki with Zucchini Chips*)
- **Eggplant** – 1 large (*Lentil and Vegetable Stuffed Eggplant*)
- **Acorn Squash** – 1 medium (*Vegetable-Stuffed Acorn Squash with Quinoa Pilaf*)
- **Carrots** – 2 medium (*Tuscan White Bean Minestrone*)
- **Onion (yellow)** – 4 medium (*Grilled Chicken and Quinoa Salad, Whole Wheat Veggie Primavera Pasta*)
- **Garlic** – 1 bulb (*Garlic and Herb Roasted Lamb with Minted Pea Puree*)

Fruits

- **Mango** – 1 large (*Quinoa Tropical Mango Coconut Porridge*)
- **Banana** – 4 medium (*Greek Yogurt Parfait with Fresh Fruits, Trail Mix Power Clusters*)
- **Blueberries** – 2 cups / 300 g (*Whole Wheat Blueberry Pancakes, Greek Yogurt Parfait with Fresh Fruits*)
- **Lemon** – 3 medium (*Herb-Crusted Baked Cod with Lemon Zest, Garlic and Dill Salmon Fillets*)
- **Orange** – 1 medium (*Citrus Kale and Orange Smoothie*)

Dairy & Alternatives

- **Parmesan Cheese (grated)** – ½ cup / 50 g (*Herbed Chicken and Farro Pilaf*)
- **Mozzarella Cheese (low-fat)** – 1 cup / 120 g (*Spinach and Artichoke Stuffed Bell Peppers*)
- **Milk (low-fat or plant-based)** – 2 cups / 480 ml (*Whole Wheat Blueberry Pancakes*)

Nuts & Seeds

- **Almonds** – ½ cup / 50 g (*Nutty Quinoa Energy Bars*)
- **Pecans** – ¼ cup / 30 g (*Steel-Cut Oat Maple Pecan Pumpkin Porridge*)
- **Flaxseeds (ground)** – ¼ cup / 25 g (*Nutty Quinoa Energy Bars*)

- **Dates (pitted)** – 1 cup / 150 g (*Almond & Date Energy Balls*)

Herbs & Spices

- **Parsley (fresh)** – 1 bunch (*Garlic and Herb Roasted Lamb with Minted Pea Puree*)
- **Mint (fresh)** – 1 bunch (*Garlic and Herb Roasted Lamb with Minted Pea Puree*)
- **Dill (fresh)** – 1 bunch (*Garlic and Dill Salmon Fillets*)
- **Paprika (ground)** – 1 tsp (*Spiced Shrimp and Vegetable Skewers*)
- **Cinnamon (ground)** – 1 tsp (*Pumpkin Spice Oatmeal Cookies*)

Grains & Legumes

- **Whole Wheat Flour** – 1 cup / 120 g (*Bran and Berry Power Pancakes, Pumpkin Spice Whole Wheat Muffins*)
- **Oats (rolled)** – 2 cups / 180 g (*Savory Spinach and Mushroom Oat Porridge, Apple Cinnamon Oat Bars, Banana Oatmeal Cookies*)
- **Barley** – 1 cup / 200 g (*Barley and Mushroom Soup*)
- **Farro** – 1 cup / 180 g (*Lemon Herb Farro Pasta Salad*)
- **Chickpeas (canned)** – 2 cans / 800 g (*Chickpea and Spinach Stuffed Peppers, Cauliflower and Chickpea Tikka Masala*)
- **Black Beans (canned)** – 2 cans / 800 g (*Black Bean and Sweet Potato Buddha Bowl, Spicy Black Bean Salsa with Whole-Grain Chips*)
- **Lentils (dry)** – 1 cup / 200 g (*Vegetable and Lentil Shepherd's Pie*)

Proteins

- **Eggs** – 12 large (*Spinach and Feta Egg White Scramble, Tomato Basil Poached Eggs, Almond Flour Lemon Waffles*)
- **Greek Yogurt (plain, unsweetened)** – 2 cups / 480 g (*Zesty Lemon Herb Tzatziki with Baked Zucchini Chips*)
- **Ground Turkey** – 1 lb / 450 g (*Maple Dijon Glazed Turkey Roulade with Cranberry Relish*)
- **Turkey Breast (boneless)** – 1 lb / 450 g (*Herb-Infused Turkey Breast with Cranberry Glaze*)
- **Tilapia Fillets** – 2 fillets / 10 oz / 280 g (*Cilantro Lime Tilapia with Steamed Asparagus*)
- **Chicken (whole or pieces)** – 1.5 lb / 700 g (*Rosemary and Garlic Roast Chicken with Root Vegetables*)
- **Trout Fillets** – 1 fillet / 8 oz / 225 g (*Paprika and Thyme Baked Trout*)

Vegetables

- **Spinach (fresh)** – 6 cups / 180 g (*Spinach and Feta Egg White Scramble, Chickpea and Spinach Stuffed Peppers, Stuffed Portobello Mushrooms with Spinach and Feta*)
- **Sweet Potatoes** – 2 medium (*Black Bean and Sweet Potato Buddha Bowl*)

- **Cauliflower (head)** – 1 medium (*Creamy Cauliflower and Broccoli Risotto, Cauliflower and Chickpea Tikka Masala*)
- **Broccoli (florets)** – 2 cups / 300 g (*Creamy Cauliflower and Broccoli Risotto*)
- **Mushrooms** – 4 cups / 400 g (*Barley and Mushroom Soup, Stuffed Portobello Mushrooms with Spinach and Feta*)
- **Zucchini** – 2 medium (*Zesty Lemon Herb Tzatziki with Baked Zucchini Chips*)
- **Asparagus** – 1 bunch (*Cilantro Lime Tilapia with Steamed Asparagus*)
- **Tomatoes (Roma or similar)** – 6 medium (*Tomato Basil Poached Eggs, Vegetable and Lentil Shepherd's Pie*)
- **Onions (yellow)** – 4 medium (*Barley and Mushroom Soup, Vegetable and Lentil Shepherd's Pie, Cauliflower and Chickpea Tikka Masala*)
- **Garlic** – 2 bulbs (*Rosemary and Garlic Roast Chicken with Root Vegetables, Zesty Lemon Herb Tzatziki with Baked Zucchini Chips*)
- **Carrots** – 2 medium (*Vegetable and Lentil Shepherd's Pie*)
- **Bell Peppers** – 2 large (*Chickpea and Spinach Stuffed Peppers*)

Fruits

- **Bananas** – 3 medium (*Banana Oatmeal Cookies*)
- **Apples (any variety)** – 2 medium (*Apple Cinnamon Oat Bars*)
- **Mixed Berries (blueberries, raspberries, or similar)** – 4 cups / 600 g (*Mixed Berry Sorbet, Mixed Berry and Flaxseed Smoothie, Bran and Berry Power Pancakes*)
- **Lemon** – 3 medium (*Zesty Lemon Herb Tzatziki with Baked Zucchini Chips, Lemon Herb Farro Pasta Salad*)
- **Raspberries (fresh or frozen)** – 1 cup / 150 g (*Raspberry Lemon Tartlets*)
- **Cranberries (fresh or frozen)** – 1 cup / 150 g (*Maple Dijon Glazed Turkey Roulade with Cranberry Relish*)

Dairy & Alternatives

- **Almond Flour** – 1 cup / 100 g (*Almond Flour Lemon Waffles*)
- **Cheddar Cheese (grated)** – ½ cup / 50 g (*Stuffed Portobello Mushrooms with Spinach and Feta*)
- **Feta Cheese (crumbled)** – 1 cup / 150 g (*Spinach and Feta Egg White Scramble, Stuffed Portobello Mushrooms with Spinach and Feta*)
- **Milk (low-fat or plant-based)** – 2 cups / 480 ml (*Bran and Berry Power Pancakes, Pumpkin Spice Whole Wheat Muffins*)
-

Nuts & Seeds

- **Almonds** – ½ cup / 50 g (*Apple Cinnamon Oat Bars*)
- **Flaxseeds (ground)** – ¼ cup / 25 g (*Mixed Berry and Flaxseed Smoothie*)

Herbs & Spices

- **Parsley (fresh)** – 1 bunch (*Herb-Infused Turkey Breast with Cranberry Glaze*)
- **Rosemary (fresh)** – 1 bunch (*Rosemary and Garlic Roast Chicken with Root Vegetables*)
- **Dill (fresh)** – 1 bunch (*Zesty Lemon Herb Tzatziki with Baked Zucchini Chips*)
- **Paprika (ground)** – 1 tsp (*Paprika and Thyme Baked Trout*)
- **Cinnamon (ground)** – 1 tsp (*Pumpkin Spice Whole Wheat Muffins*)

Grocery Shopping List for 15-21 Day Meal Plan

Grains & Legumes

- **Buckwheat Groats** – 1 cup / 200 g (*Buckwheat Blueberry Banana Nut Crunch*)
- **Quinoa** – 1 cup / 180 g (*Veggie-Packed Breakfast Quinoa Bowl*)
- **Whole Wheat Flour** – 2 cups / 240 g (*Apple Cinnamon Whole Grain Muffins, Lemon Poppy Seed Whole Wheat Scones, Cranberry Orange Whole Wheat Muffins*)
- **Barley** – 1 cup / 200 g (*Roasted Vegetable and Barley Pasta*)

- **Brown Rice** – 1 cup / 180 g (*Mushroom and Pea Brown Rice Risotto*)
- **White Beans (canned)** – 2 cans / 800 g (*Tuscan White Bean Minestrone*)
- **Chickpeas (canned)** – 2 cans / 800 g (*Moroccan Chickpea and Spinach Soup, Cauliflower and Chickpea Herb Bake*)
- **Black Beans (canned)** – 1 can / 400 g (*Chicken and Black Bean Fiesta Bowl*)

Proteins

- **Chicken Breast** – 2 fillets / 12 oz / 340 g (*Chicken and Black Bean Fiesta Bowl, Balsamic Chicken and Roasted Veggies*)
- **Pork Tenderloin** – 1 lb / 450 g (*Herb-Crusted Pork Tenderloin with Apple Cider Reduction*)
- **Salmon Fillets** – 2 fillets / 10 oz / 280 g (*Garlic and Dill Salmon Fillets*)
- **Turkey Breast (sliced)** – ½ lb / 225 g (*Lemon Garlic Turkey and Spinach Salad*)
- **Greek Yogurt (plain, unsweetened)** – 2 cups / 480 g (*Greek Yogurt Parfait with Fresh Fruits, Chia Seed Pudding with Berries*)

Vegetables

- **Spinach (fresh)** – 8 cups / 240 g (*Savory Spinach and Mushroom Crepes, Moroccan Chickpea and Spinach Soup, Spinach and Artichoke Stuffed Bell Peppers, Lemon Garlic Turkey and Spinach Salad*)
- **Mushrooms** – 5 cups / 500 g (*Savory Spinach and Mushroom Crepes, Mushroom and Spinach Whole Wheat Lasagna, Mushroom and Pea Brown Rice Risotto*)
- **Zucchini** – 2 medium (*Roasted Vegetable and Barley Pasta*)
- **Tomatoes (Roma or similar)** – 6 medium (*Spaghetti Squash with Tomato Basil and Spinach, Chicken and Black Bean Fiesta Bowl*)
- **Spaghetti Squash** – 1 medium (*Spaghetti Squash with Tomato Basil and Spinach*)
- **Cauliflower (head)** – 1 medium (*Cauliflower and Chickpea Herb Bake*)
- **Carrots** – 2 medium (*Tuscan White Bean Minestrone*)
- **Onions (yellow)** – 4 medium (*Balsamic Chicken and Roasted Veggies, Tuscan White Bean Minestrone*)
- **Garlic** – 2 bulbs (*Garlic and Dill Salmon Fillets, Herb-Crusted Pork Tenderloin with Apple Cider Reduction*)
- **Basil (fresh)** – 1 bunch (*Spaghetti Squash with Tomato Basil and Spinach*)

Fruits

- **Apples (any variety)** – 3 medium (*Apple Cinnamon Whole Grain Muffins, Spinach Apple Ginger Smoothie*)
- **Peaches** – 2 medium (*Peach and Almond Crisp*)
- **Blueberries (fresh or frozen)** – 1 cup / 150 g (*Buckwheat Blueberry Banana Nut Crunch*)
- **Raspberries (fresh or frozen)** – 1 cup / 150 g (*Chia Seed Pudding with Berries*)
- **Bananas** – 3 medium (*Banana Walnut Bread*)
- **Strawberries** – 1 cup / 150 g (*Strawberry Basil Gelée*)
- **Lemons** – 3 medium (*Lemon Garlic Turkey and Spinach Salad, Lemon Poppy Seed Whole Wheat Scones*)
- **Oranges** – 2 medium (*Cranberry Orange Whole Wheat Muffins*)
- **Cranberries (fresh or frozen)** – 1 cup / 150 g (*Cranberry Orange Whole Wheat Muffins*)

Dairy & Alternatives

- **Feta Cheese (crumbled)** – 1 cup / 150 g (*Spinach and Artichoke Stuffed Bell Peppers*)
- **Parmesan Cheese (grated)** – ½ cup / 50 g (*Mushroom and Pea Brown Rice Risotto*)
- **Milk (low-fat or plant-based)** – 2 cups / 480 ml (*Savory Spinach and Mushroom Crepes, Lemon Poppy Seed Whole Wheat Scones*)

Nuts & Seeds

- **Almonds (sliced)** – ½ cup / 50 g (*Peach and Almond Crisp*)
- **Walnuts (chopped)** – ½ cup / 50 g (*Banana Walnut Bread*)
- **Flaxseeds (ground)** – ¼ cup / 25 g (*Spinach Apple Ginger Smoothie*)

Herbs & Spices

- **Parsley (fresh)** – 1 bunch (*Garlic and Dill Salmon Fillets*)
- **Basil (fresh)** – 1 bunch (*Strawberry Basil Gelée*)
- **Rosemary (fresh)** – 1 bunch (*Herb-Crusted Pork Tenderloin with Apple Cider Reduction*)
- **Cinnamon (ground)** – 1 tsp (*Banana Walnut Bread*)

Grocery Shopping List for 22-28 Day Meal Plan

Grains & Legumes

- **Steel-Cut Oats** – 1 cup / 180 g (*Steel-Cut Oat Maple Pecan Pumpkin Porridge*)
- **Whole Wheat Flour** – 2 cups / 240 g (*Whole Wheat Blueberry Pancakes, Blueberry Almond Muffins, Lemon Poppy Seed Whole Wheat Scones*)
- **Barley** – 1 cup / 200 g (*Barley and Mushroom Soup*)
- **Farro** – 1 cup / 180 g (*Lemon Herb Farro Pasta Salad*)
- **Quinoa** – 1 cup / 180 g (*Chicken and Vegetable Quinoa*)
- **Chickpeas (canned)** – 3 cans / 1,200 g (*Chickpea and Spinach Stuffed Peppers, Moroccan Chickpea and Spinach Soup, Moroccan Vegetable and Chickpea Tart*)

Proteins

- **Eggs** – 12 large (*Mushroom and Herb Frittata, Lemon Almond Waffles, Whole Wheat Blueberry Pancakes*)
- **Greek Yogurt (plain, unsweetened)** – 2 cups / 480 g (*Greek Yogurt Parfait with Fresh Fruits, Zesty Lemon Herb Tzatziki with Baked Zucchini Chips*)
- **Chicken Breast** – 2 fillets / 12 oz / 340 g (*Chicken and Vegetable Quinoa*)
- **Pork Tenderloin** – 2 lb / 900 g (*Herb-Crusted Pork Tenderloin with Apple Cider Reduction*)
- **Lamb (boneless)** – 1 lb / 450 g (*Garlic and Herb Roasted Lamb with Minted Pea Puree*)
- **Salmon Fillets** – 2 fillets / 10 oz / 280 g (*Garlic and Dill Salmon Fillets*)

Vegetables

- **Spinach (fresh)** – 8 cups / 240 g (*Chickpea and Spinach Stuffed Peppers, Moroccan Chickpea and Spinach Soup, Spinach and Artichoke Stuffed Bell Peppers*)
- **Mushrooms** – 4 cups / 400 g (*Mushroom and Herb Frittata, Barley and Mushroom Soup*)
- **Zucchini** – 2 medium (*Zesty Lemon Herb Tzatziki with Baked Zucchini Chips*)
- **Onions (yellow)** – 4 medium (*Barley and Mushroom Soup, Moroccan Vegetable and Chickpea Tart*)
- **Carrots** – 2 medium (*Moroccan Vegetable and Chickpea Tart*)

- **Garlic** – 2 bulbs (*Garlic and Dill Salmon Fillets, Herb-Crusted Pork Tenderloin with Apple Cider Reduction*)
- **Bell Peppers (any color)** – 4 large (*Chickpea and Spinach Stuffed Peppers, Spinach and Artichoke Stuffed Bell Peppers*)

Fruits

- **Blueberries (fresh or frozen)** – 2 cups / 300 g (*Whole Wheat Blueberry Pancakes, Blueberry Almond Muffins*)
- **Mixed Berries (strawberries, raspberries, or blackberries)** – 2 cups / 300 g (*Mixed Berry Sorbet*)
- **Peaches** – 2 medium (*Peach and Almond Crisp*)
- **Lemons** – 4 medium (*Zesty Lemon Herb Tzatziki with Baked Zucchini Chips, Lemon Poppy Seed Whole Wheat Scones*)
- **Apples (any variety)** – 2 medium (*Spinach Apple Ginger Smoothie*)

Dairy & Alternatives

- **Butter (unsalted)** – ½ cup / 115 g (*Herb-Crusted Pork Tenderloin with Apple Cider Reduction*)
- **Milk (low-fat or plant-based)** – 2 cups / 480 ml (*Whole Wheat Blueberry Pancakes, Lemon Almond Waffles*)
- **Feta Cheese (crumbled)** – 1 cup / 150 g (*Spinach and Artichoke Stuffed Bell Peppers*)

Nuts & Seeds

- **Almonds (sliced)** – ½ cup / 50 g (*Peach and Almond Crisp*)
- **Pecans (chopped)** – ¼ cup / 30 g (*Steel-Cut Oat Maple Pecan Pumpkin Porridge*)
- **Chia Seeds** – ¼ cup / 30 g (*Berry and Chia Seed Breakfast Tart*)

Herbs & Spices

- **Parsley (fresh)** – 1 bunch (*Garlic and Dill Salmon Fillets*)
- **Rosemary (fresh)** – 1 bunch (*Herb-Crusted Pork Tenderloin with Apple Cider Reduction*)
- **Basil (fresh)** – 1 bunch (*Moroccan Vegetable and Chickpea Tart*)
- **Cinnamon (ground)** – 1 tsp (*Blueberry Almond Muffins*)

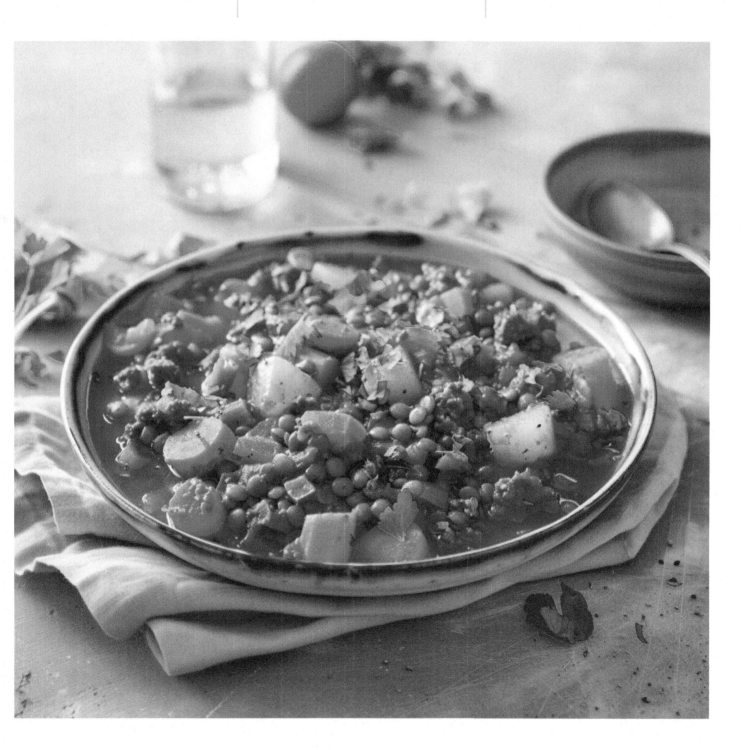

Made in the USA
Las Vegas, NV
25 January 2025

17000170R00044